The Jossey-Bass Health Series brings together the most current information and ideas in health care from the leaders in the field. Titles from the Jossey-Bass Health Series include these essential health care resources:

*Curing Health Care: New Strategies for Quality Improvement*, Donald M. Berwick, A. Blanton Godfrey, Jane Roessner

*Managed Care Contracting: A Practical Guide for Health Care Executives*, William A. Garofalo, Eve T. Horwitz, Thomas M. Reardon

*Managing Patient Expectations: The Art of Finding and Keeping Loyal Patients*, Susan Keane Baker

*New Rules: Regulation, Markets, and the Quality of American Health Care*, Troyen A. Brennan, Donald M. Berwick

*Physician Profiling: A Source Book for Health Care Administrators*, Neill F. Piland, Kerstin B. Lynam, Editors

*Profiting from Quality: Outcomes Strategies for Medical Practice*, Steven F. Isenberg, Richard E. Gliklich

*Restructuring Chronic Illness Management: Best Practices and Innovations in Team-Based Treatment*, Jon B. Christianson, Ruth A. Taylor, David J. Knutson

*Status One: Breakthroughs in High Risk Population Health Management*, Samuel Forman, Matthew Kelliher

*Strategic Leadership in Medical Groups: Navigating Your Strategic Web*, John D. Blair, Myron D. Fottler

# The New Health Partners

Stephen E. Prather
with
Thomas D. Barela
Carolyn A. Lee
Linde F. Howell

Foreword by James S. Roberts

# The New Health Partners

## Renewing the Leadership of Physician Practice

Jossey-Bass Publishers
San Francisco

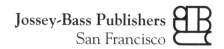

Jossey-Bass books and products are available through most bookstores. To contact Jossey-Bass directly, call (888) 378–2537, fax to (800) 605–2665, or visit our website at www.josseybass.com.

Substantial discounts on bulk quantities of Jossey-Bass books are available to corporations, professional associations, and other organizations. For details and discount information, contact the special sales department at Jossey-Bass.

 This paper is acid-free and 100 percent totally chlorine-free.

**Library of Congress Cataloging-in-Publication Data**

Prather, Stephen E.
    The new health partners : renewing the leadership of physician practice / Stephen E. Prather.
        p.   cm.
    Includes bibliographical references and index.
    ISBN 0-7879-4024-0 (hc : alk. paper)
    1. Medicine—Practice.  2. Medical care—Quality control.
3. Medical care—Cost control.  4. Leadership.  I. Title.
II. Title: Renewing the leadership of physician practice.
    [DNLM:  1. Partnership Practice—organization & administration.
2. Practice Management, Medical—organization & administration.
W92 P912n 1999]
R728.P68   1999
610'.68—dc21
DNLM/DLC
for Library of Congress                                    99-22322
                                                            CIP

FIRST EDITION
*HB Printing*   10 9 8 7 6 5 4 3 2 1

# Contents

# Foreword

Although many see nothing but storm clouds on health care's horizon, it is likely that a confluence of strong forces will reshape our field in very positive ways. The most important of these forces are

- Evidence-based care: A large and growing body of knowledge informs us about what works and doesn't work in the delivery of health care. That knowledge is readily available, and is being used, by professionals, consumers, business and government.

- Intolerance of variation: There is palpable frustration with the persistence of substantial and unjustified variation in access, costs, outcomes, and satisfaction.

- Demanding consumers: We now see the approaching wave of acute and chronic illness in a group (the baby boomers) that is used to having its needs met and, just as important, to taking an active role in health care decisions.

- The information commons: The Worldwide Web and other electronic sources have made information about health and health care easily accessible to a society increasingly comfortable with computers. This trend will shape consumer expectations and demands and force physicians to relinquish their hold on knowledge. If we are wise, we will become trusted guides, interpreters, and synthesizers.

- Systems awareness: Clinical and administrative professionals are, in impressive numbers, acknowledging the toxic effects of their historic isolation from and mistrust of each other and are finding ways to work with each other and with their customers and communities.

- Greater focus on the core business: All of these factors are forcing health professionals to become more effective in measuring, redesigning, and continuously improving the core work of our field—to prevent, cure, restore, and comfort.

Because, like politics, all health care is local, these forces will manifest themselves differently in every community. But manifest themselves they will, and the health system they create will be much different, and better, than the one we now have. Empowered by a broadly held understanding of our science and able to collect and use performance information to improve our core work, partnerships of consumers, health care professionals, and communities will reshape their local health system so that it is much better able to prevent, cure, restore, and comfort.

Competitive advantage will go to those who are both fast and focused in making this inevitable transformation, a journey that will require an experienced guide. We are fortunate to have such a guide in Stephen Prather. His unusual background, blending solid clinical experience, strong grounding in measurement and continuous improvement, and highly regarded work as an educator and consultant, makes him uniquely qualified to chart this journey for us. *The New Health Partners* not only links practical guidance to well-researched theory, but it also provides a rich array of real and fictional illustrations that helps us "get it" and see how to move from where we are to where we need to go.

Of particular help is the book's overarching framework: the "six dimensions of the new practice of medicine." Other books and a mind-numbing array of conferences and consultants focus on one or just a few of these dimensions. They either do not or cannot paint the full canvas for us—the essential interplay among structural integration, incentive alignment, process improvement, empowered teams, and partnering with the family and community. To his great credit, Stephen Prather understands and describes each of these essential activities and their interrelationship so clearly that we can also understand and apply them.

Because health care is filled with professional silos, responsibility for these six interrelated dimensions are currently divided. In largely unconnected efforts, senior leaders head integration and alignment strategies, improvement professionals guide process measurement and change initiatives, human resource departments train teams, and an array of individuals lead patient and community partnering efforts. The result of these crippling, disconnected efforts is frustration, mistrust, and, most important, systems that do not achieve their immense promise.

To correct this, everyone involved in these activities must see the link among them and follow a roadmap to the place that the powerful forces noted above are telling us we must go. *The New Health Partners* provides such a roadmap. I urge the leaders of health care systems to read and study this enlightening book together. And, since integration, alignment, improvement, teamwork, and partnering are relevant activities at all levels of an organization, it would be wise for leaders to encourage and enable the many natural work groups in their organization to also study, digest, and adapt the rich knowledge available in the pages that follow. Doing so will produce a much more effective and competitive health care system.

James S. Roberts, M.D.
Vice President—Physician Leadership
VHA, Inc.
Irving, Texas

# Preface

# Practicing Smarter Not Harder

This book evolved out of the thinking of many dedicated professionals who felt it was necessary to address the changes required by the health care dilemmas of our time. In situations that lacked physician leadership, these professionals took risks rather than observing the current system deteriorate. Getting involved in the solutions described in this book requires physicians to move forward even though uncertainty greets them at every turn. The solutions described in this book will help these courageous physicians expand their impact.

Because of the ethical dilemmas in medicine, it is impossible to prescribe a simple solution. The assumptions that influence physician behavior highlight how complex the shift to a new, more informed practice of medicine will be.

- Most physicians feel right about giving care, and patients want care to relieve their suffering.

- Most feel it is fair to pay for health care, yet not everyone can afford it.

- Physicians have been so successful at extending life that much more care will be needed in the future.

- The amount of dollars available to pay for care will be far less than the amount that is needed.

- The public is attempting to reform the current system.

- Forcing regulations and control on physicians causes resentment.

- Resentment can cloud judgment.

- Most physicians want control, but now control will come from data and a new public accountability.

- As the volume of disease treatment and unnecessary care are measured and systematically reduced, several accusations will be leveled against physicians.

- These accusations will begin to shape the overall physician response to change.

- Some physicians will be accused of wrongdoing.

- Some will be accused of overtreatment for economic gain.

- Some will be accused of withholding needed care for economic gain.

- Some will have their skills called into question as error-rate analysis gains sophistication.

- Some physicians will be singled out as best practice providers.

- Some physicians will be singled out as inadequate to practice medicine.

- The physician response to these new pressures will be driven by either fear or wisdom. There is no middle ground.

- It is easier to stay the same out of fear or indifference than it is to change out of wisdom in search of truth.

- Many physicians feel it is wrong to withhold care and to benefit economically even if the care is unnecessary.

- Though it is clear that the system provides too much care, many physicians feel no personal obligation to work toward a solution.

Humans are unique in their ability to search for truth. Although the definition of truth changes with new knowledge, this search is what directs human evolution. The force within us to search for the truth has led us to discover unprecedented ways to care for each other. To find truth we have had to readdress what is right constantly as care has become more and more sophisticated.

Medicine, society, and its physicians could not have predicted or prevented the dilemmas they currently face. They have simply set the stage for the next evolutionary step in redefining caring.

This book challenges physicians and organizational leaders at a very human level. In this climate of constant change, these individuals will either evolve or invite criticism, a process that has already begun. Physicians are being asked to rethink the path to caring. They will either build new partnerships to solve the new health care crisis or they will be accused of having caused it.

This book recognizes that although there are no easy solutions, there is a clear direction: one guided by careful observation of new information, one that shares responsibility through an innovative use of patient education and that recognizes physicians' resistance to accepting personal responsibility for a health care system in crisis. If the system can reward physicians for their integrity and build a set of structures to help them work smarter, society will benefit from a new, clearer delivery of care.

It is the sincere intent of the authors that this book stimulate those who are most dedicated to reform health care at the point of delivery.

# Mastering the Six Dimensions
## of Physician Leadership

Twentieth century medicine is quickly giving way to a twenty-first century model in which the once idealized physician-patient relationship is being eclipsed by a more accountable relationship between the physician and the public. Those who mourn the demise of the "good old days" should recognize that medicine is being challenged by the public to move beyond its own success. The modern era of discoveries and cures is no longer enough. The public has developed a whole new set of expectations that include low cost, customer service, education, and better results. This book outlines a professional and ethically sound response to unrealistically high patient expectations in an environment of rapidly increasing competition. Physicians must make monumental changes to have a successful practice. Yet the opportunity to create a physician-led delivery system rather than one driven solely by the marketplace has never been greater. If professionals respond to the challenge with a clear plan, they will gain the enviable position of leaders of the medical system. If they fail to take the steps to lead new emerging partnerships, all that has been achieved in the recent era of medical progress will be in jeopardy.

Senior adults saw medicine conquer acute disease. They had a level of expectation—to be cured—because of medicine's progress. We are standing at the beginning of a new era, one that encompasses a new science of systems thinking and information management. Because of technology, changes in medicine and public expectation will continue to accelerate. The public remains largely unaware, as do many physicians, that this new era of information will affect the world of health to the same degree that sanitation did in the 1800s. Medicine's future success will be shaped by the ability to see information quickly and the use of cause-and-effect analysis to create better health care.

Two penetrating questions have marked the collapse of the past medical era: Is more always better? Are patients getting what they pay for? The science of computerized information has finally advanced enough to answer these two questions. This has led to a new era of accountability. The data have shown that cutting the cost of disease treatment in half does not raise the morbidity or mortality rate of those receiving the care. The disturbing fact is that in some chronic diseases, as costs have gone down, the morbidity of the patients has actually been visibly reduced.

New businesses such as computer software and hardware companies, medical service companies, home health, and physician practice management companies are all growing rapidly and are helping physician practices master the new science of information-driven change. In this new era physicians must build partnerships to obtain access to the information that shows where profits can be made by delivering the best care for the least necessary cost. The skills for achieving success as a physician have changed. Accountability and fierce competition will separate those who can adapt to the new business rules of medicine from those who will refuse to change.

## General Approach

The approach described in this book ties core health care concepts together in clear cause-and-effect relationships, relationships that were impossible to see prior to the era of computer processing. Physicians can now electronically generate summaries of data about the cost and frequency of specific care steps. This new capability enables physicians to see the wide variation in care decisions and cost that results in the same good outcome. Because they can generate these data summaries themselves, physicians can also learn from themselves and avoid misinformation. By working smarter, physicians will be rewarded for using new information to guide the proven and practical approach in this book. The new measure of value compares the quality of care with the cost. To achieve the highest value of care, physicians must use a new approach.

Transforming health care delivery systems involves forming new partnerships to achieve the highest value. These new relationships will demand clear professional and ethical leadership as well as new skills. Some physicians have stepped up to guide this transformation, and they are shaping the future in the process. Others have already been left behind. Those professionals who have learned to use information, make improvements, and sustain them through sound partnerships are developing new strategies and are aggressively training each other in the skills needed to succeed. These practices are agreeing to strive toward a new expectation that defines professional "right" action in this new era of medicine. A failure to respond to today's realities will have a fatal impact on some physicians' careers.

This book describes a series of steps that will simplify the complex decisions that physicians must make and offers a roadmap to point the way for dedicated professionals. Those who undertake this journey successfully will distinguish themselves as part of the best health care delivery system. But even more important, those same professionals will be acquiring skills and using them cooperatively to transform the measurable health status of the communities they serve.

## Synopsis of Chapters

Chapter One reviews the evolution of health care that has brought society and medicine to this point. A review of the recent past clearly shows the accelerating pace of change. Medical treatment has become so technical, so successful, and so expensive that physicians face a constant series of dilemmas. Though most patients still expect a cure for everything, those who purchase care, many of them employers, cannot afford the high costs. Until the data prove otherwise, the public will continue to act on the belief that they can purchase lower cost care and still get the same good outcomes that they have come to expect. Now that a new public expectation is unfolding, the ability to use data to compare outcomes and cost is rapidly distinguishing those professionals who have learned to achieve the best practice.

In Chapter Two, the science of systems theory is simplified into usable cause-and-effect rules. The complexity of how systems work is simplified with medical examples. Understanding the medical financial systems enables the reader to see how care is being analyzed and paid for. Changing care to achieve the success described in this book follows clear cause-and-effect rules. Successful partnerships realize the importance of working together in a collaboration capable of applying these new-systems thinking skills to health care.

The cause-and-effect relationships of physicians' decisions and the flow of money are described in Chapters Three through Eight as the six dimensions of the new practice of medicine. Each of the dimensions contributes to care and reinforces each other in leading to new strategies. Physicians and their partners can use this new understanding to transform the practice of medicine for their own good as well as the community.

In Chapter Three, strategies for using information to build the integration of care across a continuum are reviewed. Chapter Four explores methods to create economic incentives to motivate physician change. Chapter Five outlines a method to implement a proven approach to clinical quality improvement. A reading list for clinical improvement science and specific clinical process improvement (CPI) and disease state management (DSM) projects is included. Chapter Six describes how these strategies can be strengthened via a high performance model that involves a host of new provider partners. In Chapter Seven, a strategy to include the family in disease state management and prevention is added. Chapter Eight provides examples of engaging the community in a new type of partnership.

In Chapter Nine, a model to support the new partnership infra-structure is introduced. An institute or data office is necessary to implement the six dimensions of the new practice of medicine. A plan to coordinate and integrate information with education and continuous communication provides the basis for an operational plan. Chapter Ten describes a method for managing the measure-ment and reward processes. Implementing good techniques to im-prove clinical practice and creating efficient office practices are shown to have an impact on disease state management. A detailed operational structure is included in this chapter that will motivate physician change.

Chapter Eleven discusses how organizing right-sized cooperative groups of physician partners can actually lessen the frequency of many expensive but manageable medical conditions. In doing so, physicians will also have a more profitable practice. Techniques such as new accounting methods, professional partnerships, and com-puterized information links can help cooperative clinical groups manage chronic diseases as well as implement innovative designs for office efficiency. This chapter explores how physicians and other caregivers can deliver profitable day-to-day care with these tools.

Chapter Twelve examines how physicians can partner with busi-ness. The winners in the new era are forging provider-business part-nerships that promote a healthier workforce by preventing unneeded physician-patient encounters. New business coalitions are already bypassing the third-party system, and physician part-nerships are taking advantage of this situation by working directly with their patients' employers.

Chapter Thirteen addresses how the approach described in this book can be used when forming community partnerships commit-ted to building community-wide health. Under this approach, patient and public education are almost as important for a physi-cian's success as advancements in treatment. By taking on roles that support the continuum of care, communities help patients benefit from physicians' efforts to manage disease.

In Chapter Fourteen, a curriculum for teaching physicians how to lead the changes that are reshaping medical care is outlined. The curriculum begins with a focused strategy to achieve the skills described in Chapters Three through Eight as the six dimensions of physician leadership. The new curriculums that are being used by successful health care partnerships across the country are helping to accelerate and sustain the new practices of medicine while also shaping the personal responsibility of coming generations.

Chapter Fifteen summarizes the critical concepts contained in this book. The final recommendations are for those readers who will build a network of physicians to accelerate a transformation of health care.

## Audience

This book is written for physician leaders who are willing to lead the new partnerships described here. With this approach they will be able to direct an ethically sound, clinically practical, and financially successful response to the rapidly changing health care environment.

Educators who teach professionals how to deliver care will find the content of this approach particularly helpful. This material can be integrated into a curriculum that unites the professions under a common philosophy to create the new practice of medicine.

Health system executives will find a strategic plan to build trust with physicians while taking advantage of the clinical improvements that are critical to the future of managed health care. The relationships among information, aligned incentives, clinical improvements, interdependent professionals, patient-focused disease management, home care, and collaborations within the community provide a blueprint to construct long-term planning.

For the practicing physician who wants to have an impact on the future of health care while achieving clinical, professional, and economic success, this book can be used as a self-study text to build the right partnerships based on the right principles to redesign medical practice.

## Acknowledgments

Many people have contributed their personal experience to this work over the past six years. Organizations that implement change through participating in one of the many Medical Resource Management (MRM) research or training programs have helped this work emerge. The physician participants in these programs, as well as those who responded to the National Integrated Medical Practices Aligned for Quality (IMPAQ) Survey of physician values and practice attitudes, have offered insights that helped clarify the need for this book.

The VHA, Inc. at the national level and VHA Southwest, both based in Texas, have provided the leadership and vision to experiment with implementing these concepts so that the transformation can evolve more quickly now, when change is so critical.

Charlotte Roberts, a long-time friend and the coauthor of the *Fifth Discipline Fieldbook*, deserves recognition as a top designer of education and consulting for learning organizations. She introduced me to systems-thinking, dialogue, and organizational learning.

Susan Corning and the Leland Kaiser family have helped bring clarity to the community issues that are a key part of this health strategy.

Brent James, at Intermountain Health Care (IHC) in Salt Lake City, is another long-time colleague and my CPI mentor. He proved to me that the technical improvement strategies in this book are not only possible but are real and working somewhere. He first educated me through many one-on-one sessions in his office and then encouraged me to integrate CPI with my work in risk management and improved physician cooperation. It was Brent who helped me see that this was the critical next step for health care reform.

Dorothy Weber of IHC contributed the critical concept of accountability and helped me see the whole system more clearly. Jackie Mead, also at IHC, provided invaluable feedback and refinement of the original CPI research design that proved that there is a link between cooperation and technical change. She helped me see the critical importance of tracking the implementation of CPI and completing simple projects before moving on.

Dick Gibson, now at the Sisters of Providence in Portland, Oregon, and Lee Steinlauf, the senior computer engineer for Medical Resource Management, refined MRM thinking about the requirements of data management for the new practice of medicine.

The entire staff at Medical Resource Management and all of the MRM consultants who have freely learned and given to each other over the last few years have created many unique and specific steps that define the strategies for new practice partnership contained here. The most significant contributors are those who have coauthored this work: Thomas D. Barela, Carolyn A. Lee, and Linde F. Howell.

Special thanks goes to the editors who have helped these ideas become a book—first to Andy Pasternack, senior health editor at Jossey-Bass, who forced me to make this book a practical tool for those who have the courage to lead this new era; to Rachel Livesey of Jossey-Bass, who refined the book further; and to Helen Hodgson, a long-time colleague and close personal friend. Helen's advice over the years has made an invaluable contribution to the concepts contained here.

Finally, I would like to thank my family, Cindy, Jack, and Robert, who have supported this work through loving me even when I have had to be a way from them too often.

*April 1999*                                Stephen E. Prather, M.D.
                                            Salt Lake City

# The Authors

*Stephen E. Prather, M.D., F.A.C.O.G.,* president of Medical Resource Management (MRM), leads a unique consulting force that assists health care organizations in obtaining cooperative physician involvement in the development of interdependent professional networks, integrated health care delivery systems, and clinical and cost improvement efforts. Dr. Prather is an expert on the impact of interdependent performance on clinical outcomes and patient satisfaction. Through Dr. Prather's leadership, MRM's contribution to VHA's National Physician Leadership Program earned MRM the 1997 VHA Partnership Award.

Dr. Prather has gained a unique perspective on physician leadership and on the complex task of mastering the many aspects of the medical encounter. As the author of *Medical Risk Management* and *Behavioral Types and the Art of Patient Management,* he is an expert on the impact of quality performance on clinical outcomes and patient satisfaction. His unique approach builds an interactive partnership between physicians and executives, which results in improved health care in the community. He uses the patient/ provider relationship as a model to clarify internal and external customer expectations within health care delivery systems.

After receiving a medical degree from the University of Kansas, Dr. Prather completed a residency in obstetrics and gynecology at the University of Utah and practiced OB/GYN for twelve years. He is a clinical assistant professor for the Department of OB/GYN at the University of Utah Health Sciences Center. He is a fellow and has served as the president of the Utah Section of the American College of Obstetricians & Gynecologists; he was also a member of the Medical Advisory Panel for the Pew Health Profession Commission at Duke University. Dr. Prather brings his extensive experience in clinical improvement research and comprehensive training for physicians to his position as president of MRM assisting hundreds of hospitals and physician practices across the country.

*Thomas D. Barela, M.D., Ph.D., F.A.A.P.*, is a board-certified pediatrician who has practiced general pediatrics and pediatric endocrinology for over fifteen years in Phoenix, Arizona. His medical practice is nationally recognized for its managed approach to the care of multiply handicapped children. Dr. Barela guided the growth of a traditional partnership of two general pediatricians to a dynamic group of ten general pediatricians and nurse practitioners who enjoy substantial economic benefits and document high-quality care. He has served as president and medical director of two large physician organizations and subsequently organized and served as founding president and medical director of a physician hospital organization that fostered physician access to all aspects of medical care finances, physician education, and development of alternative care centers. In addition to his position as senior physician consultant for Medical Resource Management, Dr. Barela serves on the faculty for the nationally recognized and award-winning VHA Physician Leadership Program and the VHA Cost Effective Physician Office Practice (CEPOP) Program.

*Carolyn A. Lee, M.H.A.*, received her master's degree in health care administration and policy in 1976. Throughout an extensive career in hospital administration she has held numerous leadership and executive management positions, including being the chief executive officer and administrator of a 241-bed acute care teaching hospital in a large metropolitan area in the southwest. Ms. Lee has acquired significant knowledge and expertise in managing various types of health care facilities and operations, including a physician/hospital organization, conducting staff training and development, and implementing managed care and risk and quality improvement services. She applies her knowledge of hospital administration, medical office practice management, and managed care operations toward the creation of cooperation-driven partnerships and strategies essential to emerging integrative systems. Using a unique assessment tool and process she developed, Ms. Lee assists physicians in understanding their leadership role in achieving the mission of these new partnerships through improved clinical and operational performance and service excellence. In addition to her position as senior consultant for Medical Resource Management, Ms. Lee serves on the faculty for the nationally recognized and award-winning VHA Physician Leadership Program.

*Linde F. Howell, M.A.*, is currently president of HealthQuest Consulting, Inc. She has initiated numerous Healthy Community projects, Community Partnerships, and other community building initiatives. Her innovative, futuristic views of community health, health care, and community member and provider responsibilities within the Healthy Community paradigm have been well recognized. She has also developed a model for community continuums for disease management including components of demand management and the inclusion of community volunteers (Community Champions). She has been involved in several Medicaid projects; working with Health Community projects that address population medicine and cultural access issues with managed care structure. Ms. Howell is also a sought-after facilitator in building organizational and community collaboratives, organizational change management, and strategic planning workshops. Before joining HealthQuest

Consultants, Inc., Ms. Howell was a director with Premier within the Center for Community Health Improvement. Ms. Howell has also served as adjunct faculty for the University of North Carolina–Chapel Hill, the University of North Carolina–Charlotte, and Pfeiffer College. She received her master's of arts degree from the University of North Carolina.

# The New Health Partners

# 1

# Serving a Changing Society

Medicine in the twentieth century has produced a series of remarkable discoveries that have significantly improved lives and increased lifespans. As a result, the American public has boundless expectations for new discoveries and cures in medicine. As we move from doctor-centered care with low regard for cost or value to a new practice of medicine that is seamless, patient-focused, and affordable, we must ensure that patient expectations more closely match the current reality.

This chapter will define the differences between the old and new medicine. The challenges of managed care, practice redesign, and disease state management all require a more innovative response to problem solving than the industrialized methods of mass production can provide. Electronic communication, high technology, access to more information, and a new understanding of partnerships are all necessities for success in this new era.

American medicine has led the world in discovery and innovation. Although physicians were trained in and utilized technical advances that made medicine widely available and more effective than ever before, they were unaware of the true cost of these wonderful innovations. The American public believed that the high cost of finding cures was more than offset by the benefits. The government also supported the effort to increase the quality of health care by creating Medicare and Medicaid. Although the working uninsured remained a serious problem for the system, the government's effort was seen as generally positive. However, progress was not made without a high price. By the 1970s, the health care system had already begun to move toward bankruptcy. Few saw the crisis coming, and even fewer responded.

Now we, as a society, face the crisis that few tried to avert. The money has run out, the population is aging, and more people are stressing the system. Universities trained too many physicians, and communities built too many hospitals. Some of the providers were paid too much. Technology made specialist jobs so complex that they could not perform their duties perfectly. The insurance industry and the government replaced charity with the third-party payer. Litigation then made it possible for the courts to award millions of dollars in damages to patients who were injured through the inadequacies of a science whose results were far from perfect or guaranteed.

Rightly or wrongly, physicians will be the focus of the effort to overhaul the system. If physicians choose an unsound method, harm will be the likely result and physicians will probably be blamed. The question is, How should physicians respond?

## The Evolution of Patients' Expectations

Before solutions are offered, let's review the evolution of patient and public expectations. For all its shortcomings, amazing advances were made in the medical era from the 1920s to 1990s. Physicians overcame most acute and infectious diseases. For most people, it is unthinkable that someone today could die from a sore throat or earache. Cuts are expected to heal. Yet many senior citizens remember the fear brought on by something as commonplace as a fever in the days before antibiotics, sophisticated surgery, computerized tomography (CT) scans, magnetic resonance imagery (MRI), and genetic engineering.

This era of medicine was profoundly influenced by two great forces: advances in medical research and industrialization. Many people benefited from the discovery of antibiotics and other drugs, but the wide availability of these drugs was possible because of the industrial mass production of pharmaceuticals, sterile equipment, new anesthetics, medical supplies, and immunoserums. Because of its dependence on new medical discoveries, the multibillion dollar pharmaceutical industry drove most medical progress. Medical schools educated their students to use the miraculous new tools. The industrialization of pharmaceutical companies, medical suppliers, and hospitals made these miraculous new tools widely available (Ackerknecht, 1982).

## Creating the Cures

Prior to the industrial scientific era, the real objective of medicine was to diagnose and explain diseases that could not actually be controlled or cured. Physicians knew more about the consequences of disease than anyone else did, but they had few tools to change outcomes significantly. Physicians learned that microbes caused disease, but they couldn't figure out how to kill them. Each discovery was a step forward, but most of these "magic bullets," as they were called, were toxic. Salvarsan, the chemical therapy for syphilis, killed the bacteria but the therapeutic range was so close to the lethal dose that it could leave the patient injured or worse.

The modern era of medicine that paved the way for the new practice of medicine described in this book was marked by a series of key events. One of these occurred in 1923 when Sir Frederick Grant Banting and John James Richard Macleod shared the Nobel Prize for discovering insulin. Scientists began to see that diseases were associated with specific failing organs. In diabetes, these were the pancreas and end organ receptors for insulin. Banting and Macleod proved that the hormone insulin could be extracted from an animal's pancreas, sterilized, and injected into humans to save their lives.

Eli Lilly took this key discovery and began a rapid expansion made possible by the power of American industry. By mass producing the products of scientific discovery, Lilly went on to become the pharmaceutical giant that it is today. Medical discoveries would have done little more than make for interesting journal articles without the ability to mass-produce products consistently.

In many ways Banting and Macleod's discovery and the new medically focused businesses that would use industrial techniques to develop scientific findings marked the turning point that led to the modern medical era. Interestingly, the practicing physicians of this time did not believe in the industrial concepts of production. They retained a guild mentality with an emphasis on personal authority and mentorships in education. They did not try to decrease their variation in care to attain the high consistency that made other health care businesses a success. They saw their role as a professional, not a businessperson.

Medical discoveries and the consistent production of drugs like antibiotics were leading the way to the modern era even though physicians were not pressed to make their practices efficient or consistent. Medicine was turning from an art to a science. Physicians discovered how the body worked and then learned to fix whatever was broken. Medical cures were discovered faster in the next few decades because of new technology, business, government, and philanthropic support (Sidel and Sidel, 1984, p. 131).

Penicillin launched physicians into the true era of mass treatment. Penicillin, along with sulfonamide, changed the course of World War II. For the first time in history, more soldiers died from direct warfare than from disease. Penicillin was the magic cure the public had hoped for. Now Americans would see the real pharmaceutical industry emerge, and society could, for the first time, imagine a world without disease. The discovery of medical cures accelerated after World War II (Burnham, 1982, pp. 1474–1479).

Organ-specific cures were discovered in the 1940s and 1950s. Suddenly acute disease was being turned back in less than a generation. Human society and its expectations of medicine would never be the same. The public dreamed that physicians would eliminate or cure all disease.

This public expectation was reinforced by the discovery of Salk's polio vaccine in 1955. This remarkable discovery became the standard by which society would measure the efficacy of all medicines, because this vaccine, along with the Sabin vaccine that followed, was able to completely eliminate a dreaded killer.

### Rising Expectations

Following the eradication of polio, the public stopped dreaming about cures and began to expect them. The press began to cover medicine's progress, making high profile media heroes out of new surgical wizards like Michael E. Debakey and Denton Cooley, who could reconstruct the arteries of the heart. Surgical transplant superstars replaced organs that had failed. The public expected medicine to bring them total cures. The possibilities seemed endless. The public wanted and got more, and it was all driven by scientific discovery and a business strategy to sell the tools of the medical trade.

In recent years, the progress of medical research has been so rapid that it has been almost impossible to track (Star, 1982). The advances that became widespread usually made a profit for some business. The free enterprise economy and the marketplace determined what technology would be mass-produced following scientific research. Tax dollars and marketplace economic forces shaped the sale of these technologies. Competing companies selected research that demonstrated the value of the equipment, drug, or procedure that would sell their product. The products then gave physicians the opportunity to put the discoveries to good use. Most of these new, high-tech solutions were delivered at a higher price than the procedures they replaced. In all of the progress of medicine, the public barely noticed the gigantic profitable businesses that were shaping access to their care.

The market forces of the 1950s and 1960s included the third-party payer. Once Medicare and Medicaid were firmly in place, medicine appeared to be free for the majority of the population. This illusion created by the third-party payers caused spending to accelerate even more, until the result was an obvious financial strain on the American economy (Scofea, 1994, p. 3).

## The New Practice of Medicine

To survive in this new era of health care, physicians must commit to change. While building on the success of modern medicine, physicians need to master a whole new set of skills to thrive in this new health care environment. I call this confluence of past medical success and new realities the *new practice of medicine*. The new practice of medicine consists of a compulsive system of recording, reporting, and rewarding the actions of physicians. This book details the steps necessary to operationalize high performance, continuous improvement, and a reward system for the delivery of best care. The new practice uses information not only to communicate but also to decide which processes need changing. With this information, physicians can create business partnerships that can reward them for their contribution. As summaries of outcome and cost data become more widely disseminated, patients will seek out these types of practices.

This type of information is already available to the savvy and technologically adept consumer. For example, the Internet already publishes individual physician mortality and cost statistics that consumers can access directly via their personal computers (Williams, Nash, and Goldfarb, 1991, pp. 810–815). Many local and national newspapers regularly publish utilization comparisons of hospitals and physicians as well.

Hospitals use data to boost market share by establishing themselves as "the best"; this means someone else is the worst. These types of comparisons have begun to force new physician behavior. For the first time in the evolution of medical care, physicians across a single specialty are embracing a uniform and consistent approach to best practice when treating a single disease. Cardiology and the approach to congestive failure, and cardiovascular surgery and the treatment of coronary artery disease, provide excellent examples (Hannan and others, 1994, pp. 761–766).

The elements of the new practice of medicine include

- clear analysis and reporting of data

- reward

- practice improvement

- high performance

- disease state management

- patient education

- community partnerships

With the goal of improved care, professionals from across the health care continuum are working together for the first time in the new practice of medicine. These interdependent professionals define and consistently deliver the highest quality of care at the lowest necessary cost. They also maintain high patient satisfaction with full access and low risk of liability. Most important, professionals in the new practice are confident that they have not harmed patient health in their efforts to economize. This challenge to do no harm is no longer a formidable one because of the wealth of information that surrounds us.

For those who are prepared, there are hidden opportunities and benefits to be found in this health care crisis. For example, the economic pressures to lower reimbursement will create an opportunity to improve the quality of care. Because purchasers of care are usually either a business or the government, they are interested in buying the least expensive care. Therefore, the practices that can achieve the lowest cost will be attractive to the purchasers of care. With the proper measurement of outcomes, decreased variation in care, and a clear understanding of process and outcome relationships, practices can achieve economy without decreasing quality (Eddy, 1994, pp. 817–824). Without good information or the knowledge of how to use it, there is concern that physicians will respond to financial pressure by eroding the quality of care.

Be assured, the pressure to economize will have an impact on physicians. Practices will begin to separate themselves into two groups. Practices in one will achieve success because they lower cost and consistently get better outcomes. Practices in the other group will experience worse outcomes as a result of the pressure to keep costs down. Those who are prepared to improve care through the structure and strategy described here will separate themselves from those who miss the opportunity.

### Rationing Care

One popular strategy accepts that harm is a risk traded for the opportunity to make dollars under a system that is committed only to preserving the bottom line. Under this model, rationing health care is the means to higher profits. Aware of this strategy, the public fears that their health care is inadequate. In response, patients are using information as a weapon and filing lawsuits against rationing practices that cause patient harm. In one lawsuit, a family in California successfully sued a physician who had refused to order a mammogram for the wife, who was the mother of two children, because of restrictive managed care guidelines. She later died of a cancer that had gone undiagnosed for too long.

Although lawsuits are becoming more common, most people don't have the resources to carry out a lawsuit. However, legislative action offers another remedy. A concerned public is demanding a patient bill of rights. Professional organizations such as the National Patient Safety Foundation of the American Medical Association have promised to focus attention on physician errors (Goldsmith, 1997, p. 1561). Patients are holding physicians and hospitals accountable for any harm that appears to have occurred as a result of cost cutting. This new level of scrutiny is beginning to separate physicians who are prepared from those who risk a patient's well-being to cut costs.

## Taking a Path Less Traveled

There is another, more ethically sound, alternative to rationing care. It is defined by the new practice of medicine. With this approach, physicians predict success based on changing care by using cause-and-effect analysis instead of by rationing care. The patients are actually given the tools to take responsibility for prevention and disease management. Several types of partnerships are necessary to create this new practice of medicine. These partnerships include professionals providing care at the practice level, hospitals, and other facilities. In addition, partnerships are needed with all the businesses that contract, purchase, and sell medical services.

The new practice of medicine will provide important economic incentives. Thanks to computerized data systems, it is easy to see who is making an economic contribution to the delivery of care, who is costing too much, and who is making a profit. With increased access to data, physicians can clearly see the economic impact of specific clinical changes. As information about real cost becomes more accessible, pressure for changes will increase. For example, many business coalitions have discovered that non-value-added third-party services could be eliminated, thus saving specific dollars as they go to the contracting table (Halvorson, 1993, p. 120).

## The Influence of the Community

Communities—for example, New York City—are taking on a new role in health care. The New York City Health and Hospitals Corporation is the city's public hospital system. Because of the data being collected by public health officials, they are able to set performance standards for the medical schools that have students training in the New York system (Perlman, 1991). Well-organized, committed groups of people in communities are beginning to influence the systems of medical care that they depend on. Further examples will be detailed in Chapter Thirteen.

New partnerships will face many challenges in implementing the new practice of medicine. They will have to create cooperation among people who have traditionally been disconnected. All partnership organizations, including providers, must share information and build common strategies. If they fail to define responsibility and accountability, they will find themselves in conflict.

Choosing between the strategies of rationing or integrated cooperation boils down to one central question: Are those providing the new practice of medicine willing and able to learn new skills in order to change? The prospect of learning new skills can be a daunting one to physicians already scared by the tumultuous health care environment. But these new types of partnerships between physicians and organizations are succeeding by replacing denial with determination. They are managing this by building new relationships and new infrastructures focused on using information cooperatively. Physicians are learning to use information to answer critical questions rather than relying on old assumptions.

## Using Information in a New Way

New partnerships must first determine what the community wants, and then create a plan to cut costs. To implement change, groups of providers within the partnership strategy must utilize information in a coordinated, cooperative, and compulsive manner. Physicians at the forefront of this new strategy use computerized information and Internet technology to help them see the cause-and-effect results of making certain decisions.

### Computerized Information

By using computerized clinical and financial reports, physicians can clearly see their impact on the bottom line. For example, a group of hospitals partnered with the commitment to share what they learned as they installed a computerized clinical and financial reporting system. As a result, the physicians were able to create a monthly report on the results of disease state management. This report also showed the impact on each physician's income. Using facts and clear, timely reports, these physicians formed a users group to help each other redesign care at the point of implementation. With this reporting effort, physicians discovered that the data clearly showed that an old approach was failing. Physicians could see in reports linking clinical failure to economic impact that holding onto old behaviors was a disadvantage. With solid proof that income was being adversely affected, the physicians were supportive of implementing new processes.

Another group practice was able to use this type of analysis and reporting when they faced the dual challenge of having an oversupply of physicians coupled with a rapid decline in reimbursement. Because they were a small, cohesive group, the physicians could agree on issues such as cross coverage, wages, and data collection, and they were able to create personal reports. This practice decided to create a plan to redesign the delivery of care. They began by establishing the key indicators they wanted in their report. Next, they began using education and aggressive disease management. Their hospital gave them cost and quality analysis reports that showed the number of unnecessary hospital days occurring within their patient population. They used their data to project how much the overutilization costs were and how much they would save by decreasing hospital days. Studying the reports, the physicians discovered a dilemma: To save the money spent on these patients, including their own fees, there was a cost added to the practice with no reward. In fact, they found that fee-for-service was penalizing them financially. The analysis and reports also demonstrated what the impact on their incomes would have been if they had been able to keep a portion of the savings created through risk sharing under a fixed budget. The message that they were losing money that they had saved for the insurance company was the impetus to change.

Because facts opened the physicians' eyes to just how much reward they could have shared under new shared-risk partnerships, they decided to form a new practice.

Reports and data will not resolve all dilemmas. In fact, shifting to risk sharing through partnerships usually creates new dilemmas. One such dilemma is, "My success now depends on our success," or "If you fail, I could fail." The only sure success within cooperative partnerships is to ensure that your partners succeed. While the correct facts and analysis are helpful, more than anything physicians need high level communication and a common business strategy to survive in the new practice.

*Internet Technology*

The Internet, telemedicine, interactive computers, CD-ROMs, and diagnostic centers at the workplace are all part of the new practice of medicine. By using these new support systems, a practice can create savings for whoever sets the budget to pay for care.

The Internet and other advanced telecommunications devices link doctors with a community and provide them with almost instant access to a wealth of information. Scottsdale Memorial Hospital is building an Intranet with fiber optic links into an 8,000–unit community development. This new commitment to communication is planned as a strategy to pay off as better compliance with home care decreases utilization. The result of making access to medical advice easier is better health. New medical group practices will help these communities decide how to manage their data as well as participate in high-quality care. Practices that embrace this technology view patients as partners in the battle against disease and help patients use prevention to improve their health throughout their lives.

## Putting the New Practice into Action

Phoenix Pediatrics in Phoenix, Arizona, offers a classic example of operationalizing the new practice strategy. (This example will be further expanded in Chapter Eleven.) Responding to rapidly decreasing reimbursement, these physicians developed a new method to manage a population of multiply handicapped children. Under a risk-sharing medical contract with the state, the physicians used home-care and outpatient settings for their clients. Practices employing a risk-sharing medical contract are given a budget to cover total expected costs. If Phoenix Pediatrics could provide care for less than the budget, they could profit. But if their costs exceeded the budget, they were at risk for the loss. The practice needed to develop protocols, triage systems, and a partnership for cooperative care with the families of these children in order to minimize their risk. Because they were able to keep their patients healthy, they were able to keep part of the savings they created. For the opportunity to create a profit, they were willing to take the risk that real costs might exceed their budget. Phoenix Pediatrics used facts to track utilization before and after new practice protocols went into place, and their financial forecasting and communication paid off. Not only were they able to keep part of the savings they created, but they also improved the quality of care. They predicted that they would succeed because the cost of partnering with the children's families through education was far less than the savings achieved by keeping them out of the hospital. The children were healthier, the families were happier, and the physicians were able to profit while proving that they had a positive impact on the patients they served. These professionals practiced the new medicine and reaped the rewards.

## Building New Competencies

Practicing doctors and health care executives need a specific and ongoing curriculum to thrive in an ever-changing environment. Health care educators are beginning to teach the competencies needed to find new solutions. These core competencies include business principles, managed-care strategies, new partnership requirements, and techniques to use information for learning.

Educators are simultaneously advancing the notion that providers will assist patients with self-diagnosis and disease prevention. The Healthcare Forum's Healthier Communities Summit and the Institute for Healthcare Improvement (IHI) provide information and ideas for professionals who are educating their patients. Every year the new practice of medicine described in this book grows in importance at these events. With an educational focus and a formal curriculum, the new practice of medicine can be reproduced community by community. The following skills are some of the core competencies of a curriculum for the new practice of medicine:

- Evidence-based medicine

- Population-based analysis

- Business management

- Protocol implementation

- Patient and family care mapping

- Home-based education and protocol tracking

- Disease state management cooperation with communities

- Self-care and self-diagnosis

The recipients of care, directed by these new skills, learn techniques that help them manage their own diseases and health by working with a variety of providers.

### Achieving the Deeper Reward

Through this curriculum, the new partnerships reward their patients by helping them achieve maximum benefits from their system of care. More practices are adopting this approach because the personal rewards are even greater than the economic savings.

The diabetic patient is an example of personal rewards for the new practice. If all diabetic patients had their blood sugars managed aggressively, a recent study projected that it would add 920,000 years of life free from blindness. It would eliminate many amputations and cases of renal failure. It would also add 611,000 years to diabetic patients' lives overall (Diabetes Control and Complications Trial Research Group, 1996, pp. 1409–1415). Naturally, the short-term economic success of shortened hospital days is also of value. However, saving and improving patients' lives is surely the greater reward for the involved health care professional.

Through education, patients have the opportunity of increasing their self-awareness and well-being. Education also gives physicians the chance to build new relationships with patients and create deeper personal understanding of prevention through education, thereby decreasing the frequency of disease. But who will teach physicians to educate patients?

### The Need for Teachers

Education for providers is critical. Assessing the physicians' attitude and knowledge is important to curricular design. Different approaches will be needed for all types of learners. The selection of teachers is also critical; they must have the credibility as well as the skills to help their peers analyze their own success and failure. Some physicians will be unable to achieve disease state management goals, even if the system only rewards those who succeed. This is likely to create resentment and resistance to learning. The teachers of this new curriculum must teach a method of change even when the providers fight against it. Only through a successful change management program will providers be able to implement the new practice of medicine.

The key challenge facing educators will be to help the physician move from the industrial era's model, "work harder," to the new era's model, "work smarter by using information." Successful integrated partnerships are focusing on the latter model. These groups are gaining an understanding of cooperative performance, the flow of money, and linking cost to care. They are also building opportunities for new community partnerships.

Anyone interested in implementing the new practice must first learn about systems-thinking and address the key steps of cause-and-effect analysis as practiced by today's most progressive health care organizations. The ability to see the consequences of actions and reactions provides the cornerstone for all that follows.

With this foundation in place, the next chapter will explain how physicians can identify simple systems within highly complex organizations. Reinforcing and balancing systems of cause and effect, the challenges of delay, unintended consequences, and the creation of intended results are all reviewed. Accountability is shaped by these principles, and information defines the results achieved by partnerships committed to accountability.

# 2

# Making Systems Work

This chapter explores the concept of systems thinking. Examples drawn from the health care environment illustrate the complexity of systems and the predictability of change. Although it is often thought to have its roots in engineering, systems theory is modeled after biologic observations (Von Bertalanffy, 1968). Systems theory is eminently adaptable and can be applied to any clear, measurable set of actions and reactions (Paich, 1985, pp. 126–132). This systems approach has been used to design cities, organize massive business enterprises, and predict the future (Forrester, 1961).

In systems thinking, complexity consists of a collection of discrete simple systems. The impact of actions in terms of the reactions they cause is measurable and predictable in each distinct system (Senge, 1990, pp. 68–126). Using this logical systems, thinking physicians can manage the complex challenges facing them. By agreeing on what can be safely changed via a systematic approach, physicians can organize into groups of providers with a common strategy.

The most common system archetypes that physicians are using in response to the economic pressures of the health care crisis are covered in this chapter. Human behavior, clinical care, and business structures all contain some simple systems that follow systems thinking laws. To achieve the massive cooperation necessary to implement the new practice of medicine, physicians in a partnership need to identify these simple systems and use systems thinking to organize the information.

## Systems Thinking and Information

Systems thinking allows physicians in new partnerships to find a balance between what they do, what they want, and what the real results are. When physicians manage disease in populations with plentiful and accurate data and clear goals, physicians can utilize systems thinking to predict outcomes and economic impact. Systems thinking enables physicians to see the cause-and-effect relationship of facts within the care they provide and the partnerships they create. In the past, physicians often relied on assumptions that were not supported by facts. This type of thinking should be replaced by a systematic review of the data. Most physicians work with dedication, good judgment, and common sense, but until recently they didn't have access to the information that clarified simple cause-and-effect relationships within the complex health care system.

Without access to data, physicians focused on their patients' short-term crisis. This tendency to treat the symptoms rather than the cause has its roots in traditional medical training and organizational distrust and complexity. For example, when a chronically ill patient returns over and over again with pulmonary or cardiac complaints, a physician's natural response is to treat the symptoms. With systems analysis, physicians can predict the long-term cost consequences of repetitive treatment and suggest a formal intervention designed to stop the need to treat. The cost of education, home health, and tracking the patient's participation are weighed against the decreased cost of treatment. When the calculations predict both a positive patient benefit and cost savings, the new approach should be implemented. Additional measurement is used to track whether the system solution continues to work. To sustain the gains, partnerships also need to reward themselves for changes that result in cost savings.

Community leaders expect more from health care providers than simply treating the short-term symptoms of patients and advising them to return for more advice or care. We now have proof that educating patients to care for themselves actually decreases the need for physician time (Cohan, Pimm, and Jude, 1991). Cutting-edge physician partnerships are leading the change from the old style of medical practices to the new practice by following systems thinking. These physicians are assessing, implementing, and then measuring the care they provide. Based on predictable cause-and-effect relationships among cost, treatment, education, and recovery from illness they are constructing a new strategy to improve care and cut costs.

Before computerized information, it was impossible to see the impact of medicine on a population. As a result, both good and bad practices went unrecognized. For example, early extubation after bypass surgery was done in some locations for years before population-based comparisons showed its benefit. Now it is accepted practice—failure to use it is seen as indirectly causing harm. The systems thinking approach compares the frequency of other procedures being done in similar populations. This has led informed physicians to decrease total hip replacement, coronary artery bypass grafts, and hysterectomies (Center for the Evaluative Clinical Sciences, 1996). Systems thinking can prove what works and what doesn't.

The power of systems thinking is that it helps physicians recognize that the best solution for a single patient isn't the most appropriate remedy for the entire population being served. For example, a patient with multiple, vague complaints goes from doctor to doctor for more and more care until a complication occurs in a treatment that was moderately helpful at best. If the result of care for these patients can be summarized in a report that links treatments to outcomes, it becomes clear why these patients are cost outliers. With a new commitment to communication of such information, physicians can identify who these patients are and what care is not likely to work.

## Systems Theory and Business Structures

Because the impact of the complex relationships among all of the components of care are measurable, we must use systems thinking. One reason is that malpractice cases follow a model of systems theory. For example, a hospital hired temporary nurses to cover swings in volume in the intensive care unit (ICU) to cut down on costs. One temporary nurse didn't know where to find the equipment that the physician needed to place a central venous catheter to monitor blood pressure in a very ill patient. The physician found himself in the middle of a minor procedure with unfamiliar tools, and a major complication was the result. The administrative decision to use temporary staff in the ICU was the beginning of the system's failure, but the lawsuit focused on the failure of the physician. Any decision that cuts costs at the expense of patient safety is a system failure. New partnerships track errors and look for the root causes behind system failures. They use systems thinking to eliminate problems as they redesign the way they practice.

One possible solution to the previous ICU example would be to simplify the wide variation in technique used by the physicians. A uniform approach often simplifies the complexity of medical care. The error that actually caused the patient injury could be blamed on the hospital, but the physicians in this example had a better solution. If the cause of the error was the wrong equipment, they tried to determine why multiple sets of equipment were being stocked for the same procedure. By using only one set of equipment for this particular procedure, the potential for this error is eliminated. Cause-and-effect analysis is needed to explore the links between the actions of one part of the system and the reaction in another part. This is not crisis management—it is prospective tracking of key indicators of quality failure.

Systems thinking applied to the business side of medicine can expose short-term strategies that are fundamentally flawed. For example, the temptation of immediate reward has made it difficult for large insurance companies and HMOs to think about long-term strategies. The absence of long-term thinking explains why prevention is not usually covered by policies, even though it would ensure more long-term gain from a systems perspective.

A critical success factor for the new practice of medicine is to help professionals overcome their tendency to depend on short-sighted action. Physicians only need to understand the basics of how systematic cause-and-effect cycles work to create the outcomes that will ensure success.

As actions are taken, their impact can be illustrated with arrows that are getting either smaller or larger (see Figure 2.1). These arrows represent the link between actions and reactions. Some cycles reinforce actions, some balance or resist actions, but all actions have consequences.

One type of cause-and-effect cycle is called the reinforcing loop. As illustrated in Figure 2.1, an action stimulates a reaction that, in turn, stimulates the initial action. The reinforced action then reinforces the reaction in an eternal cycle. All of the arrows in this system move in the same direction, and all get progressively larger. Because this simple system is interconnected, each reaction is dependent on change in some other part of the system. In a reinforcing loop, action is always affected by the reaction. An example of a reinforcing loop would be a new medical practice that grows as its reputation builds. This growth brings the opportunity to see more patients, which builds a better reputation, which enlarges the practice further.

Barring any outside constraints, the reinforcing loop continually increases as each side of the interaction reinforces the other.

**Figure 2.1. The Reinforcing Loop.**

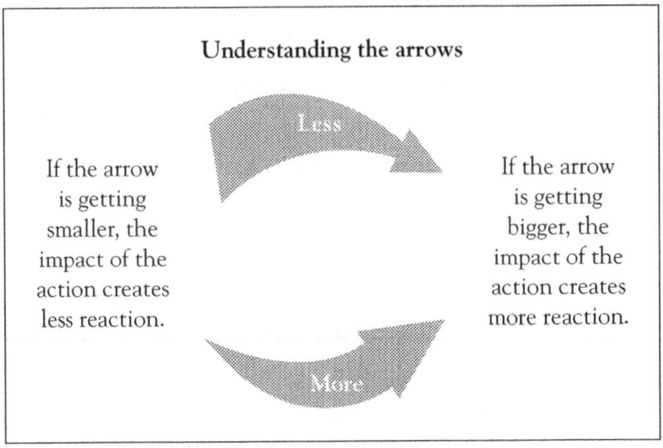

Consider a savings account or any other investment whereby interest is automatically reinvested. This type of account is an example of a reinforcing loop (as shown in Figure 2.2). The deposit draws interest, thus adding to the principle. It then draws even more interest, which then creates a larger reinvestment and principle. Withdrawing part or all of the principle will, of course, end the effectiveness of the reinforcing loop.

Finding health "interest" wherever it exists and reinvesting part of it to create more principle is a basic concept behind the success of the new practice of medicine. (In this discussion the words *interest* and *savings* are used in a purely economic sense.) Organizations in the growing partnerships that deliver care should not withdraw all the savings they create as they decrease the need for medical care. When the third-party payer (insurance) chooses to remove all the savings that the new partnerships created, either through distributing it to stockholders or by acquiring more businesses, it threatens the entire system. Reinvestment of savings to create the needed rev-

Figure 2.2. The Positive Reinforcing Loop.

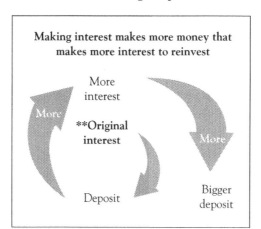

enue to cover future health care needs is a systems-thinking approach to preparing for the aging population. If the gains in one part of the system are continually removed or sacrificed to another part of the system, the possibility of reinvestment for the future is lost. The new practice of medicine constantly reinvests in information systems, new practice support, and continuing education.

### The Negative Reinforcing Loop

Keep in mind that not all reinforcing systems achieve positive interest. Some reinforcing cycles have a negative impact. For example, when an elderly patient gets ill, medicine provides care, resolving the problem, thus leading to a longer life. This leads to the need for even more care, which prolongs the life even further. Carried out with no reinvestment strategy, this approach to care will bankrupt the system. Whether or not we have the resources to care for our aging population is dependent on systematic reinvestment in the new practice of medicine.

### The Balancing Loop

Another cause-and-effect cycle is the balancing loop (see Figure 2.3). It often exists in opposition to a reinforcing loop. In a balancing loop, a positive action causes a reaction that tends to buffer the system or return it to its normal state. A good example is the thyroid.

Low thyroid levels stimulate TSH, which stimulates the thyroid to secrete more T4. As the thyroid level increases to normal, the TSH drops and the stimulus slows down. If the thyroid stops responding to the TSH levels, the hypothyroidism TSH levels remain high until thyroxin is administered. As serum T4 levels go up and return to normal, TSH levels also become normal. Understanding what conditions affect which part of this balancing loop enables physicians to identify the proper therapy and predict outcome. The success or failure of a treatment can be analyzed based on balancing biologic relationships.

The balancing loop concept helps simplify our understanding of physiology and endocrinology, although by gross oversimplification.

**Figure 2.3. The Balancing Loop.**

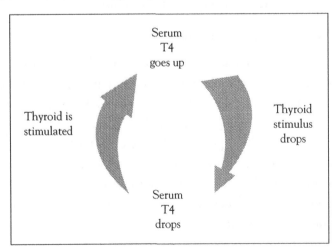

By simplifying a complex process into generalizations, physicians can take actions and review outcomes at a summary level. Physicians do not need to understand the detailed molecular biology or even the details of biophysiology of many human systems, but they must learn the shorthand model of balancing systems and recognize when an expected result does not occur. Although this concept may appear simplistic, consider how many loops a physician has to track in many different patients in a single day. The practice of medicine is dependent on simplifications, trials of care, and evaluation of results via systems thinking. Because the human body is a classic example of multiple concurrent balancing loops, care is often planned at a simple system level.

Another example of the balancing loop is the body's response to hunger. The normal response to hunger is to eat until the stomach is extended, at which point one no longer feels hungry. However, stress can cause an individual to snack all day, thus leading to obesity, a significant health problem. Prevention can focus on eliminating stress by building habits that lower stress and counter overeating. But if patients ignore their own cause-and-effect feedback by over-reacting to stress, they can make themselves very sick. In fact, at least 50 percent of medical care is for disease that the patients themselves could have prevented (Goleman and Gurin, 1993, p. 17). The new practice approach uses the balancing loop model to predict the impact of a wide variety of care options. Some physicians recognize that when patients are sick, medicine doesn't necessarily represent the only treatment.

Physicians can also teach patients to use the mind to heal. The patient's neurophysiology or healing ability is complex, but if the results are generalized into action-and-reaction systems, it becomes possible to observe the results of educational interventions. The body carries out a very important balancing act of cause and effect within the immune system and the reticular activating system. If successful, education gives patients new possibilities to find "interest" within what is referred to as mind-body medicine. In other words, education teaches patients that if they "invest" in their own health, they will reap their own "health interest" (Goleman and Gurin, 1993, p. 39). This mind-body link as a balancing system can be used in powerful ways. For instance, for individuals to end their harmful addictions, they can be helped to find will power to improve their own health without medication. By formalizing social support for these patients, the new practice can save on medical treatment costs.

The issue of patient compliance illustrates the complexity that exists in even the simplest patient care scenario. A patient with a chronic illness is part of the system. To maintain health, the patient must comply with the medical plan by being seen periodically. This is a balancing loop. Care is given until the desired results are achieved, thus suggesting that no more care is needed. Patients understand that if this care maintenance step is left out, their health will get worse and at some point they might need hospitalization. The current system usually does not remind patients about care maintenance. Because patients want to stay healthy, in most instances they will check their own medication and follow a plan for good health. However, this desired patient response requires motivation and knowledge on the part of the patient. Therefore, part of care for the new practice of medicine is emotional support for patients.

By ignoring these balancing loops, physicians run the risk that a medical treatment will fail, thus resulting in the need for very expensive recovery therapy. For example, an acute episode such as a myocardial infarction cannot always be fixed by going back to preventative care. Once enough of the myocardium is damaged, even bypass surgery won't restore the heart.

## The Challenge for Organizations

The challenge for health care organizations is to focus on a solution before a crisis, not after. Sometimes saving one part of the health care system is not enough. Neglect may have already caused other key systems to collapse. For example, many integrated health care

systems have been ignoring the negative impact of decreasing revenue in practices that are successfully lowering the need for care
through disease state management. Once physicians have lost revenue unfairly, it can be nearly impossible to rebuild the trust needed
to work together. The solution is to try to predict the impact on
income before new actions are taken.

### Improving Care

Partnerships should devote themselves to the goals of fairness and
achieving the best possible outcomes. To have an impact on many
preventable diseases, partnerships need to add alerting systems. Just
as patients need a reminder to take their medications properly,
providers also benefit from this type of support. The new alerting
mechanisms are called *decision support,* and when tied to formal
efforts to achieve clinical process improvement (CPI), they give the
practice a tremendous advantage. When these alerts are tied to education, they can be powerful tools. If a medical condition such as
renal failure occurs due to drug toxicity that has advanced too far
before the drug is stopped, recovery requires more medical treatment
than should have been needed. The more damaged the physiological system, the more expensive it is to fix. The cost of recovering
from iatrogenic injury is measurable and can be contrasted to the
cost of prevention via alerts and decision support. When the cost of
prevention in a large population is lower than the cost of treating
the injury, these savings are recoverable.

Decision support as a strategy to decrease costs and improve care
before it causes complications has been refined (and in many cases
pioneered) at Intermountain Health Care (IHC) in Salt Lake City,
Utah. The University of Utah School of Medicine, Department of
Medical Informatics, and IHC, under the leadership of medical information management experts Homer Warner, Reed Gardner, John
Evans, Stan Pestotnik, and others, have raised the standard of thinking about medical decision making (Millenson, 1997, pp. 80–89).

By creating reminders and order options that prevent errors of omission or overtreatment, IHC has been able to improve outcomes dramatically (Classen and others, 1991, pp. 2847–2851). Reminders give providers an awareness of real patient needs rather than waiting for complications to get everyone's attention. By showing physicians new information prior to the complication, they are able to make decisions that prevent iatrogenic injury.

IHC's pharmacy management tools, linked to the laboratory, use cause-and-effect analysis to predict the results of medical decisions based on past experience. The tools advise the physicians on drug choice before the patient experiences a poor result from exposure to the wrong drug or drug dose. If the decision being suggested (the action) is not likely to get the desired result (the reaction), the electronic medical alert asks the physician if he or she would like to consider another option. At Latter Day Saints Hospital, when a patient gets an infection of a specific organ, the physician can quickly find out which organisms have cultured out of similar patients with the same type of infection. The electronic medical alert also contains information about the bacteria's antibiotic sensitivities (Pestotnik and others, 1996, pp. 884–890).

At the time of prescription, the physician in a matter of moments can choose the least costly drug that has the highest sensitivity in like circumstances in that hospital and on that floor. A few years ago, prior to server technology, use of systems thinking to analyze cause-and-effect relationships required a megacomputer system such as IHC's HELP system. Now, however, these decision support models are being put on PCs. This technology will make it easier for physicians to make quick, accurate decisions. By using reminders and seeing the facts behind therapeutic reinforcing and balancing loops, a new understanding of what works is beginning to change physician behavior and practice patterns. The outcomes are redefining the potential of medical care. By measuring units of care as actions and then measuring the reaction linked to unit-based cost, the desired cost outcome can also be achieved by design. This use of systems thinking makes it possible for millions of dollars to be saved and reinvested in future systems-thinking strategies for success.

A formal effort to help the chronically ill break old habits is a classic new partnership strategy. New information, reminders, and education help patients help themselves. This approach helps empower patients who are capable of decreasing their need for care, thus allowing the physicians to divert more time and energy to prevention and education and so help the patients even more.

### Seeing Unintended Consequences

Using information and systems thinking, physicians are able to define process steps that are inadvertently causing problems for patients. By recognizing these problems as unintended consequences that are predictable and by examining the cause, it becomes possible to systematically remove them. The practice then establishes a new care plan that pays off in terms of disease state management.

In the new practice of medicine, care providers search for the unintended consequences that predictably occur from old, independent, disconnected medical processes. Poorly coordinated quality of care is still the norm in many locations. When physicians have never been shown the connections between process and outcome, poorly coordinated care is the result. Now that it is possible to measure many clinical results such as disease recurrence or unplanned readmissions, the public is beginning to make direct comparisons of providers. They usually focus on unintended consequences of the physician's or hospital's actions. For example, retreatment of preventable injuries, and the expected incidence of injuries from treatments that have a known risk of complications, are being measured in many locations (Leape, 1994, 1851–1857). As physicians study these unintended consequences, they achieve overall improvements that become the new national norms. Physicians that don't look at the data and fail to manage the preventable complications will compare poorly to other practices.

The power of systems thinking linked with new data makes it possible for the new practice to see what is causing specific health problems—even when the problem is an unintended consequence of earlier care. Often, well-intended care triggers a bigger problem. For example, the first-time drug reaction to a dose of an indicated drug is an unintended consequence with which all physicians must cope. Additional dollars are needed to solve this type of problem, even though it can't be avoided. However, systems thinking predicts that the second time this drug is given will represent a preventable error with both health and cost consequences. With computerized tools and alerts, the physician's ability to prevent this type of error comes closer to perfection. Improving care in the new practice means removing process errors and the complications that used to be called "the expected risk" of a treatment.

### Systems Approach to Removing Unintended Consequences

The systems laws of cause and effect provide a clear way to remove many unintended consequences of care. For example, research has shown that giving an antibiotic to a patient after a clean-contaminated surgery has a beneficial effect on recovery. When the simple step of taking this antibiotic is delayed, serious infection can occur (Classen and others, 1992, pp. 281–286). When infection occurs, all the intensive care in the world might not save the patient from a septic postoperative course, or even death. In the new partnerships that are emerging, the patients are educated and involved as part of the care team and understand their role in this cause-and-effect system. Patients expect to get an antibiotic two hours prior to surgery. If someone forgets it, they can alert a provider to the problem.

An even better system solution would follow the example set by Latter Day Saints Hospital whereby a CPI process ensures that the patient gets the drug on time, 98 percent of the time. By flagging the charts and following standing orders on clean-contaminated cases, a team of personnel use computerized alerts to ensure almost perfect delivery of the antibiotic. The result of this compulsive systematic approach to improved care has helped establish a postoperative infection rate that is five times lower than the national average (Classen and others, 1992, p. 286). Even hospitals without a strong technologic infrastructure have duplicated this model by simply making it a requirement for the operating room nurse to notify the physician exactly when the drug is given prior to surgery. By tracking the success of this process step until it is performed perfectly, the unintended complication of infection is dramatically lowered.

### Simplifying the Practice's Point of View

To achieve success, physicians must agree on what they want from the new practice. Working backwards from that vision, they must ensure that their actions fit in the chain of cause-and-effect events needed for a system of best care. This can be achieved by simplifying all the complexities of care into a series of major steps that can be thought of as a flow operating under cause-and-effect rules. Starting with the goal to keep patients well, the new practice can view a flow of all the options. For example, when the patients are ill with tonsillitis, otitis, or pneumonia but the illness presents as a cold, the new practice requires the addition of some "if, then" steps to assist the clinical decisions. Specifically "if" symptoms include fever, red throat, painful cough, or abdominal pain, "then" the practice would decide that these patients need to have someone look at their throat, possibly run a culture, listen to their lungs, examine their abdomen, or do some lab tests. Triage protocols can be put in place to guide the patient to the right provider and the right care.

But what if the patient has a sore throat, low-grade fever, and stuffy nose, followed by a cough, then laryngitis? In the next week or so the symptoms will be gone, and this condition doesn't require antibiotics or even a doctor, for that matter. The patient or caretaker would, however, benefit from education, over-the-counter drugs, and reassurance. This time the triage protocol guides the patient to an educational resource. Similar examples can be found in every specialty in which evaluating minor symptoms, although organ specific, is not a wise use of a specialist's time. Pain management provides a good example. In the new practice, physicians develop protocols to manage pain specialty by specialty.

Once patients are educated about their role in their own health care, they are far less likely to insist on appointments with their physicians or to demand overtreatment. Patients are taught to contribute to their own health future, and that behavior saves money. Kaiser of Northern California was one of the first organizations to prove this point. They changed utilization by creating telephone-advice systems and formal patient education.

### The Challenge of Delay

When everyone within the entire system masters the interrelationships among triage, self-care, health, education, community support, and medical care, the new practice of medicine is succeeding. The problem is that this mastery is sometimes difficult to achieve.

One of the skills that emerges through a study of systems thinking is the ability to see that there is often delay between cause-and-effect cycles. Because delay keeps needed data away from those responsible to act, individuals often assume they have not done enough. Because they cannot see the impact of their actions, they continue going in one direction much longer than they should. Because they don't anticipate delay, they actually cause a new problem by overreacting.

This concept can be seen clearly in how hot and cold water work in a house. Imagine trying to get hot water to the second-floor bathroom of an old house. When first turned on, cold water comes out of the hot-water faucet. The natural response is to turn on more hot water, an overreaction. When it is a perfect temperature the bather can get in, but in seconds it will be too hot. Jumping out and turning the hot water way down is overreacting again. This time when it is warm again, the bather will hop back in the shower, only to find that the temperature will go back to ice cold. It isn't until the bather understands that the problem is overreaction with the faucets that it becomes possible to adjust for the effect of the slow response time. The same metaphor applies to health care reimbursement. Because the negative impact of continuing to practice in the old fee-for-service model has been delayed, most physicians just keep working harder, failing to recognize that they are about to be "scalded." If physicians were to project the repercussions of continuing to accept deeper discounts, they would see it makes sense to shift to the new practice strategy instead of just working harder.

The best medical care also depends on understanding delay and cause and effect. Physicians predict the consequences of treatment by allowing for the delayed physiological response to a medication. For example, a reproductive endocrinologist sees a patient with a unique problem such as infertility, which was actually caused by another doctor's overreaction. A high-dose, prolonged treatment of dysfunctional uterine bleeding with hormonal suppression can cause chronic anovulation. A lower dose drug could have worked, but because the symptoms didn't resolve immediately, the first physician kept increasing the dose. When the bleeding finally came under control, the physician assumed that the high dose needed to be maintained. After years of overtreatment, the patient's normal hormonal cycles shut down. Because of the physician's overreaction when faced by a delayed response to treatment, the patient developed an expensive and frustrating infertility problem. If a complication occurs during treatment of this new condition, the second doctor may be blamed, even though the real problem was the prolonged and excessive medical treatment that caused the secondary condition in the first place.

Another example of overreaction because of delay includes patient compliance. If patients are not educated to wait a set amount of time for a course of treatment to work, they may overreact by switching treatments. For example, a patient who takes steroids for arthritis often experiences no immediate relief because the effect against inflammation is delayed. After two days, the pain is still there, so the patient goes to a psychic healer who convinces her that she will soon be well. The next day the patient finally feels better as the steroids begin to work. She credits the healer, so she stops the medicine. Several days later, when the drug is out of the patient's system, the pain returns because the inflammation is back. The patient has no way of knowing whether the drug or the psychic caused her pain to disappear. The patient has confused the issue by trying two solutions without giving either the time to work. The patient should have been educated to expect a delayed benefit. Without the patient's understanding of cause, effect, and delay, the needed time for compliance is lost.

### Use Small Work Groups for Systems Thinking

Critical to the successful use of systems thinking is the ability to respond to new facts in an organized way. The practical issue of establishing a small interdependent group of physicians that can use these tools is addressed in detail in Chapter Ten. These groups must be small enough to govern themselves with cooperation, but large enough to see significant change as they manage care. The ideal size is three to seven physicians (with their employees). Building new accountability requires a group that can see the results of care systematically. They need to be able to agree to a flow of care and then reward themselves for success. Lumping physicians together in large groups does give them a larger database and helps them achieve greater market share. The down side is that creating large groups can defeat the power of systems thinking as competition replaces cooperation. With physicians, conflict increases when groups of more than ten or twelve try to come together. Small functional groups must develop the skills to use cause-and-effect analysis prior to several of these groups' joining together. With a common commitment, they may account for hundreds of members of an independent physicians association, but the functional work groups must remain small.

### Thinking as Logical Partners

The method of seeing and then using cause-and-effect analysis requires that a core group of physicians define the logical steps that they need to take to achieve their goals. Systems thinking also requires that physicians are shown the results of their actions regularly so they can decide whether they are getting the results they actually want. This logical but compulsive approach also gives well-organized physicians the confidence they need to empower patients as they take on more responsibility for their own care. Measuring cause and effect is required as patients participate more fully in the self-care solutions that new patient education offers.

The current health care system has been using a reactive, short-term, illness-focused decision-making model that has ignored some of the predictable cause-and-effect results of prevention, education, and disease management. This occurred because incentives for practices to get organized were lacking and because the benefits couldn't be documented prior to the information era. The new, integrated health care partnerships help patients see more deeply into the chain of processes that make up their care. The system supports patients by helping them prevent illness or recover from illness when it can't be prevented.

This chapter has described a critical thought process that will help guide the new practice as it attempts to meet the future health care requirements of a changing society. In the next six chapters, the new practice of medicine is broken down into six specific systems that reinforce each other as new strategies are put in place. All the stakeholders who will create partnerships can benefit from a mastery of these six dimensions of the new practice of medicine. The next six chapters present an overview of how these key dimensions can be managed. Subsequent chapters further refine the concrete steps that organizations, including the doctors' offices, can take to support each other. The partnerships that can make these critical reinforcing systems work together will reform health care in America.

# The Six Dimensions
# of Physician Leadership

Thus far we have examined the challenges that face physicians and suggested that physicians can use systems thinking to build a new strategy for success. This chapter introduces the six key dimensions that constitute complex health care systems. These six dimensions consist of a series of reinforcing cause-and-effect process areas (see Figure 3.1). Implementing these processes will enable physicians to set clear goals, thereby ensuring their future health. Each dimension contains a series of action steps that will result in thriving practices. Each dimension is covered in the next five chapters. The six dimensions are

- integrated information exchange
- aligned incentives
- clinical process improvement
- high-performance teams
- partnering with the family
- partnering with the community

## Outlining the Core Competencies
## Needed for the New Practice of Medicine

The first dimension, integrated information exchange, should be implemented in every organization that affects care. The integration

**Figure 3.1. The Six Dimensions of the New Practice of Medicine.**

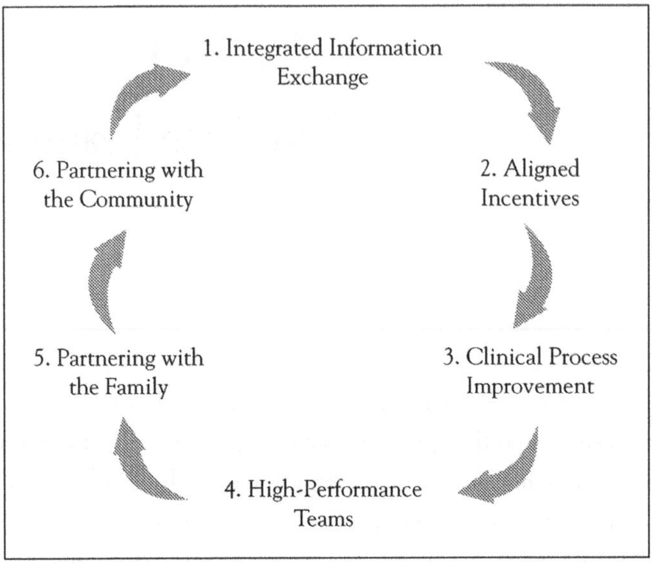

1. Integrated Information
Exchange

6. Partnering with
the Community

2. Aligned
Incentives

5. Partnering with
the Family

3. Clinical Process
Improvement

4. High-Performance
Teams

of information requires a new use of both clinical and financial data to communicate and answer discrete questions necessary to guide change. This chapter highlights techniques that use information to decrease competition and wasted efforts occurring in every part of the system. The second dimension, aligned incentives, rewards the behavior that drives the most effective approach to managing the continuum of care. Once the first two dimensions (integrated information exchange and aligned incentives) are in place, it is possible to move to the third dimension, clinical process improvement (CPI), to motivate participation. Once process indicators are measured and a system is in place to assist improvement strategies, practices are ready to move on to the fourth dimension, high-performance teams. Medical Resource Management's experience in risk management has proven that cooperative relationships accelerate the implementation of clinical improvement by eliminating errors and malpractice claims. Making improvement and cooperation an operational requirement of the partnership overcomes the physician's resistance to getting involved. The fifth and sixth dimensions, partnering with the family and community, complete the cycle. Taken in total, these six dimensions are transformative, but many organizations have had limited or even negative experiences with one or more of these dimensions.

This book will assist the new health care partnerships that have become mired in one of these dimensions and are unable to move their organizations to the next level. Some organizations have been defeated in their effort to integrate the first dimension, and remain confused by their own information or their inability to organize meaningful data. Organizations at this stage need to agree on a way to stop waste and duplication through the use of analysis and improved communication.

Other organizations are unable to move past the second dimension (aligned incentives) because they fail to recognize the value of motivating physicians economically to improve care. The failure to align incentives has left some organizations without the means to help physicians reduce overtreatment or prevent medical errors. For these organizations, the third dimension, clinical process improvement, remains elusive. Without motivated physicians, data and reports still will not lead to the positive outcomes experienced by other organizations. Lacking a method to report the right data as feedback, these organizations cannot establish needed education and process improvement.

Organizations that are unable to make the transition to the fourth dimension need to overcome negative physician behavior. Infighting and controlling behavior are often the barriers to high-level performance of the partnership. Sometimes it is the fifth dimension, providing new education to patients and their families, that remains unrewarded or underdeveloped. If the previous four dimensions are not solidly in place, most practices rarely set aside a budget to take self-care into the home. Finally, partnerships need to take full advantage of medical resources by partnering successfully with the community. For many partnerships, the sixth dimension remains unattainable. By following the strategies in this book, partnerships will be able to break the impasse by focusing on techniques to master each dimension.

The first step in the process is to master the power of information. That is, using the right information, at the right time, to answer the right questions. The remainder of this chapter focuses on the first dimension, integrated information exchange.

## The First Dimension, Integrated Information Exchange: Using Information to Integrate Across the Continuum of Care

The key word in this dimension is *information*. Integrated systems are defined by the ability to use information to link key partners within the system.

Information can only be understood and used systemwide if it is communicated properly. Information must be separated into its various components and managed via cause-and-effect analysis.

### The New Era

The new information era is in constant flux—technology advances rapidly. Fortunately, this has resulted in low start-up costs for the type of technology needed by most partnerships. Most personal computers (PCs) available on the market today can run sophisticated graphic applications. In addition, it is now standard for PCs to contain high-speed internal modems that enable users to connect to the Internet. The Internet, a computer based, on-line information source, once reserved for the government and universities, is now a multibillion-dollar worldwide center of information and commerce. Connection to this world, known as the Worldwide Web, costs under $20 per month for unlimited access. An Internet service provider (ISP) connects computer users with the Internet. America On-Line (AOL) is the biggest and most widely recognized ISP.

Computer users can now share data, video, and voice on the same telephone line. It is increasingly easy and cost-effective for partnerships to use technology to process data and communicate. Many management initiatives have been stymied because physicians refuse to embrace technology. The rapid evolution of the industry and the consequent unfamiliarity that follows new technological innovation are partly to blame. Two or three years ago, many physicians were unable to access the information they needed from their information systems departments because on-line reporting was too time intensive and cost prohibitive to implement. However, these obstacles no longer exist. The cost of the technology is affordable for almost all partnerships. The challenge today is less about measurement and more about understanding what information will create an entirely new level of communication. In the new practice, physicians use the right information to answer specific questions that will change behavior, thus making it possible to ask new questions and create the new medicine.

The barriers to using information in this new way are primarily the difficulties in changing the user's mindset and demystifying information sciences. Information systems managers need to keep abreast of technological developments and have the ability to translate technological language into layman's terms. The use of focused information embracing new technology to communicate solutions has become critical to survival, yet some fear changing to the more flexible, real-time systems. The new health care partnerships must overcome these mindsets and embrace technology. The power of integrating data is not volume, it's selection and the ability to sort and report. The new partnerships have the technology to get needed information in real time, to make informed decisions based on that information, and to create specific strategies based on facts, not assumptions. As a result of this capability, the new partnerships are able to make the adjustments in care that simply were not possible a few years ago.

## Using the New Technology

Even though information technology has matured to a point that it can organize and make medical data usable, the data must still be fed into a computer. The only data that is usable is data that can be coded. The next problem is that not all the data are important, so the providers must agree on a data selection process. This process is detailed as a key step for improvement projects in Chapter Five. The analysis process is also dependent on the hardware and software that are available (Shortell and others, 1996, p. 164). Software reports and user interfaces need to be clear and user friendly. Clinical process improvement (CPI), the third dimension, represents a tested approach that uses data to prompt a higher level of clinical performance. The new partnership must create a mindset that believes the new improvement literature published in nearly sixty quality-related health care journals. They must then blend improvement results with financial data to define operational effectiveness. The next step is to link the cost and quality data together around specific projects. This challenge requires business logic to be added to the partnership strategy. The formulas for business success require software applications that are user friendly and allow forecasts to be made at every level of the new partnerships.

## Enhanced Communication Strategies

The most important competency for achieving successful integration is sending, receiving, seeing, and believing the new data. This process is complicated because the physician/receiver of the data is often suspicious of data in general. Because old quality assurance (QA) data were often flawed, many physicians have become wary of all information. The new partnerships should place a special emphasis on gaining physicians' acceptance of the data that clarify change. The experience of professionals conducting CPI projects in hospitals across the country reinforces the importance of getting physicians' acceptance. These project leaders ran up against physicians who held onto old assumptions even when good theory showed the value of taking a new direction, thereby almost killing the CPI movement. A formal strategy is needed for clearly communicating results so that facts overcome physicians' suspicion of data.

## The Rule of Fives: Informed Communication

This solution to a widespread denial phenomenon evolved out of the hands-on experience of Medical Resource Management (MRM) faculty. These leaders couldn't understand why obvious successes achieved elsewhere did not seem to impress many of the physicians who heard the lessons. They identified the problem as a resistance to change coupled with poor communication. The solution that evolved is called the *rule of fives*. Our experience shows that if economic incentives are not driving physician participation in quality improvement projects, it takes five improvement successes in a row to shift the individual physician's mindset. Each success must then be communicated in five different ways to each physician that the partnership is trying to influence. Here are the five methods of communication that we've found to be the most effective.

1. *Educate everyone to use the new technology.* The first and most important method of communication is making the data accessible through on-line technology. But first, physicians need to be educated to access the Internet and various other forms of computer-supported reports. Then they must become comfortable and confident in doing so. For example, a group of radiologists decided they wanted to lead the improvement efforts within their integrated system. They knew that time lost in reading, rereading, and transferring x-rays had a real effect on their incomes and also introduced errors and discrepancies. Because the improvement itself required the physicians to consider viewing digitized images on a television monitor screen, it made sense for them to learn how to call up the image on both laptop and home computers. The quality improvement consultant

who organized this project began by gathering all the radiologists in a room with laptop computers. One by one each physician was taught to turn the computer on and access e-mail. Next, they were taught to send messages and receive files. Finally, they were taught to access the Internet through a website and to use a search tool to find a particular topic. Within this one-day program, the radiologists learned to enter data, find new information, and download databases into data management software tools that could print graphics such as statistical process control (SPC) charts, bar graphs, and histograms. Before physicians buy in to information technology, they need to be educated in using the technology. This step is absolutely essential.

2. *Communicate through physician leaders.* Another effective method uses physicians who are already benefitting from the changes to spread the word. For instance, a respected physician leader could approach an individual physician who has improved data with a hand shake, a word of congratulations, and a question such as, "How can you and I get more of your peers to follow your excellent example?" It is important to have a responsive strategy in place that can actually attempt to help this individual get the message out.

3. *Use graphics and other visuals to highlight results.* A report with a graphic display of the success should be widely available to key groups of people who should be coming together as partners across the continuum. Special groups of physicians inside the system are a good target for this type of communication. The departments that had input to the success should be thanked in context with the reports of results. This is done in a formal effort to create a new expectation to see results visually. This visual recognition step facilitates understanding.

A graphic display of results can be presented at meetings using PowerPoint, a laptop computer, and a liquid crystal display (LCD) panel or projector. Take time in the meeting to point out, discuss, and formally recognize each success. Asking physician champions to explain how they succeeded will lead other physicians to the conclusion that they should get more involved. This broadens the likelihood that change will be sustained.

4. *Peer-to-peer presentations.* The fourth level of communication in the rule of fives is to ask the successful physicians to present their cases and results at hospital and group practice business meetings, again making use of one or two graphics. This peer-to-peer communication of success can be organized to resemble "grand rounds." The project leaders take pride in their accomplishments, as do those who can gather their own data, thus demonstrating that a new benchmark has been achieved inside their practice. In addition, each presentation should make clear the financial impact each success has had on the organization.

5. *Add graphic representations of success to newsletters.* Although the newsletter remains the most common form of communication in most practices, it is in many ways the least effective. Clear graphics are necessary if the newsletter is to have any impact (Cleveland, 1994, p. 6). For example, a picture showing a line that is going up as it moves to the right over time offers clear visual proof of success. By adding upper and lower control limits you have a statistical process control (SPC) chart. Once physicians see this trend, they will probably look for more detailed information in the legend. Even if the data concern a different specialty, a graphic leaves an impression. Two positive graphs on the same page are even more effective, but adding more than that serves only to confuse most readers.

### Information Sharing

Sharing information is an essential ingredient for integrating the organizations needed to succeed in the new practice of medicine. Sharing information also offers the greatest challenge: Because physicians have never had to share data, resistance is often extreme. The challenge is greater still if physicians within the new partnerships are not computer literate. Physicians need to realize that without adequate knowledge of how to access information and use new computerized communications technology, they simply will not succeed. As physi-cians in the partnership increase their technology skills, those who remain independent and unwilling to share data will be uninformed, and eventually will be weeded out by the marketplace.

The focus needs to shift from very well-managed time to very well-managed patient care. To make this shift partnerships need to use information and communication between providers in new ways. Providers also need to look at the improvements that result when new actions are implemented. When physicians create their own success, it helps them overcome their natural resistance to change. The partnership is responsible for enabling providers to build an entirely new approach to care based on information shar-ing and continuous improvement.

For example, one integrated system met the challenge of shar-ing information across a continuum of providers by holding short, frequent meetings to review the significance of findings that were coming out of specific efforts to manage disease states. Those in-volved in the data sharing were educators, primary care physicians, specialists, nurses, and hospital personnel staff and administrators—all the partnership stakeholders. In meetings, presenters used clear graphic displays of significant variation in improvement of outcomes that showed before and after comparisons. The SPC charts show-ing variation over time clearly illustrated the improvement goals of the system. By sharing data, physicians are able to track the success of best practice protocols.

### Success at a Glance Evidence (SAGE™)

Information sharing has never been easier to achieve, as demon-strated by the rapid evolution of the next generation of confiden-tial, clinical, and financial reporting tools. For example, SAGE™ is a tool that Medical Resource Management (MRM) developed. It is a classic example of user-friendly, Microsoft Windows-based (object-oriented) software engineering applied to the greatest challenge that faces physicians—communication. After extensive experience watching physicians disengage with improvement efforts, it became clear to MRM that the task of sorting and computing existing data until a clear message could be generated had become a requirement for physician participation in change agendas. Physicians who need to see clear messages or trends regularly in order to be sure it is safe to change care are creating a new demand. Physicians need a tool to re-port their success or failure on a regular basis so they can reach con-sensus regarding their goals. They are motivated by seeing results that they understand. SAGE™ reports make it possible for physicians to see a few results at a glance, such as the percentage of clinical and financial goals achieved, bonuses earned, and productivity-to-wage ratios. These parameters are as important for solo-practitioners as for large group practices, but different groups need different reports if high-level communication is to be achieved.

SAGE™ reports like that shown in Figure 3.2 demonstrate the trends important to a specific group of physicians in a format they designed. Economic issues, such as bonuses achieved, are always important to physicians, and because these reports aid in commu-nication, they help sustain new, positive change. Trends on the decline provide a wake-up call. Physicians need to be able to see the results that lead to success or failure. Upon demand the reports need to show the next level of detail.

The reporting of data is rapidly being raised to an art form. Jim Frankfort, a practicing pulmonologist in San Jose, California, helped Medical Resource Management design a series of detailed comput-erized reports in specific information areas needed for the successful tracking of disease state management (DSM). The report in Fig-ure 3.3 compares the percentage of implementation of protocols, per-centage of satisfactory data entry, and clinical outcome trends to the details of specific proven clinical process steps critical to the success of DSM. The trends can easily be tested for statistical validity. The next level of detail displays the individual data as a statistical process control chart compared to peers. This type of interactive tool teaches the provider what the facts prove about the success or failure of care

**Figure 3.2. Sample SAGE™ Bonus Report.**

> **Success at a Glance Evidence**
> *Confidential Detail Report of DSM: Asthma*
>
> For: Individual Physician Code 273633
> Re: Personal Data

| Month | Percentage Maximum Bonus Earned | P < .05 |
|:-----:|:-------------------------------:|:-------:|
| 6/97  | 0   | * |
| 7/97  | 0   | * |
| 8/97  | 0   | * |
| 9/97  | 0   | * |
| 10/97 | 15  | * |
| 11/97 | 30  | * |
| 12/97 | 85  | * |
| 1/98  | 97  |   |
| 2/98  | 89  |   |
| 3/98  | 100 |   |

Average number of asthmatics
  followed = 55
Average percentage of practice = 5%
Participant since 6/1/96
Date of this report: 3/12/98

• This is a measure of the percentage of the maximum bonus achievable that you earned.

• Note: p < .05 compared to benchmark value of 100%.
Trend analysis shows a significant increase in bonus achieved.

**Percentage of Maximum Monthly Bonus Earned**
**Program start date: 6/1/97**

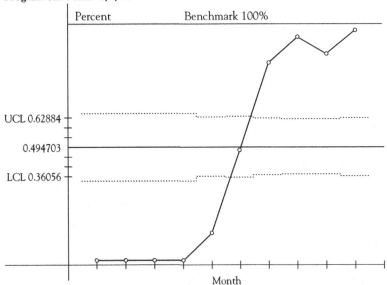

This report is a detail of bonuses earned over a ten-month period. It shows percentage of possible earnings rather than dollars in the table and uses text to explain the number of patients as a raw number and percentage of practice. The trend chart at the bottom of the page shows the significance of a rapidly increasing bonus.

at the process level. It is important to keep this data confidential, and it must be well-managed to achieve improvement. Data use is continually being refined, thus increasing the chance for success for physicians who take advantage of data management software.

As physicians learn to trust each other and begin to share data, real, substantive change happens. For instance, if one physician in a group practice achieves 90 percent of her clinical goals and makes 90 percent of the highest potential revenue, two things begin to happen. Those who are less successful begin exploring ways to improve, and those who are already successful find the data reassuring enough to sustain their best practice. Physicians who are successful as measured by the data are held up as models, and the other physicians in the practice are encouraged to follow the new practices. In addition, the partnership takes advantage of an individual physician's success by making them teachers and strategizers for the future success of their group.

### Using New Reports Systemwide

This type of clinical report can be integrated into the systemwide contracting and compensation strategies of the new practice partnerships. The success-at-a-glance concept needs to approach trends regarding financial success with the same degree of detail as the previous example. The key to using information is to start with summary data reports that are constructed from more detailed data. At a glance, all of the key players need to see the overview that is important to them in a few "bullets." If all is well, the user of the data will move on. If a trend shows surprising success or the frustration of declining success, the individual or group leader needs to be able to probe deeper, learn more, and consider change. The real power of these new reporting tools is only achieved if those who use them can find the answers they need to manage the change process. It doesn't matter how good the hammer is if there is no carpenter wielding it. The same holds true of the new electronic tools for decision support.

**Figure 3.3. Sample SAGE™ Detail Report.**

---

**Success at a Glance Evidence**
*Confidential Detail Report of DSM: Asthma Feb. '98*

For: Individual Physician Code 273633
Re: Personal Data

---

Average number of asthmatics followed = 55.
Average percentage of practice = 5%. Participant since 6/1/96.

| Outcome | Your Result | PAQ Result | Benchmark Result | Comp PAQ | Comp Bench |
|---|---|---|---|---|---|
| % DSM goals met | 90 | 70 | 100 | + | − |
| Cost savings | 2,900 | 2,000 | 3.250 | + | − |
| % proper data submission | 85 | 75 | 100 | + | − |
| Incentive bonus | 725 | 627 | | + | − |
| % max bonus available | 85 | 70 | 100 | | |
| Wage inpact (%) | 5.2 | 3.8 | | | |

Statistics: + indicates statistically greater
— indicates statistically less than comparison group

**Outcome and Measure Relative Values**

Note: The graph above shows your results for Asthma Disease Management. Outcomes compared to the benchmark and other physicians' practicing in PAQs. Statistical comparisons are located in the table above.

This report shows a breakdown of success criteria for an individual physician. The first column describes the indicator as a percentage achieved value. The second column shows the percentage achieved by the PAQ (working physician group). The third column is the benchmark result. The final two columns indicate statistical significance compared to the PAQ or the benchmark.

A good example of linking the tools with the training to become a clinical improvement "carpenter" was seen at VHA, Inc. in recent years. The strategy behind the development of physician leadership education evolved under the direction of Jim Roberts, senior vice president of VHA. Education of physicians started a process that co-evolved with the SAGE™ reporting tool and new findings, leading to new education. As a result of surveying thousands of physicians in the course of education and then using the results of assessment to design needed solutions, faculty were able to redesign ongoing education. The newly trained and inspired physicians actually designed the core logic of SAGE™ by defining the indicators of their success. Knowing what was needed for success focused new data reporting, which directed new education and continuous redesign. As SAGE™ continued to evolve, summary reports were constructed from more detailed reports, and new computer engineering was used to calculate, contrast, and compare productivity, clinical outcomes, satisfaction, and financial impact. Because SAGE™ coevolved with education, it became the perfect structure to implement and track success strategies. The physicians changed in response to the data because physicians themselves designed the reports. Most physicians who resist the data have found that off-the-shelf software is not suitable to their particular needs. Involving physicians in the coevolution of SAGE™ was a strategy that epitomizes the new practice of medicine.

### Finding Visible Fairness

In the new practice, trust means open access to data. And success can be achieved only by fostering this trust. In our experience, physician-hospital conflict is rooted in the belief that the other side has an unfair advantage. Conflict usually revolves around the issues of money, power, or the perception of unfair advantage.

To overcome distrust, all the contributors who hope to achieve economic fairness are linked under a common reimbursement strategy. When a network that shares information decides to compute the flow of money between the key contributors, physicians will note instances of visible fairness or unfairness. This new awareness guides the change process. To achieve this awareness, information systems, even those at the beginning stages, must establish outpatient and inpatient measures of medical cost and utilization. Unit-based cost tracking at the specific care level is critical to achieving visible fairness as specific changes contributed by one group or another are quantified in dollars and cents. Physicians can overcome distrust by proving that enhancing the flow of care will reward those involved in making changes.

Computing the relationship of cost and reimbursement requires complete data. Patients must be assigned a common identification number as they cross the continuum of care. Through patient identification, physicians can analyze patient need and see the benefits gained as the patient moves from the home to the office, to the hospital, to the outpatient facility, and back to the home. The expectation that multiple groups within the partnership will be guided either by the data directly or by someone trusted to interpret the flow of clinical and cost data should be established.

Clear, usable data and measures are difficult to maintain because of rapid changes in the reimbursement environment. Nevertheless, physicians need clear regular reports on the economic impact of contracts that pay for the care they provide. Without these reports, physicians cannot see the results of their actions and will see little reason to change. The new physician leaders will use facts to analyze clinical processes as they improve the continuum of care. These leaders will also use facts to resolve disagreements in a continuous effort to show stakeholders they are being treated fairly.

This chapter has focused on the power of information to affect physician behavior. If information is shared and reported across integrated organizations, the organizations can build on trust and accessibility to create a cooperative and supportive environment. The following list recaps the competencies needed to master this first dimension, integrated information exchange:

## Critical Elements for Informed Integration

- Develop a practical understanding of technology.

- Build a network link between key providers.

- Use a uniform method of data display across the system.

- Organize the current sources of data to aid communication by using the rule of fives: Get five successes and communicate the results five ways.

- Focus data collection and reporting on specific simple issues and begin reporting results.

- Help physicians overcome computer phobia.

- Use e-mail between the key organizations.

- Teach classes on Internet and electronic communication literacy.

- Build and use a website.

- Formally share data in clear, user-friendly reports across key organizations, including physicians'.

- Utilize facts to create visible fairness.

- Track what happens to the practices' income with clinical improvement and keep the records open.

- Prove that redundancy in the delivery of care is being removed.

- Display results and hold discussions to ensure that changes are seen as fair.

- Recognize the dilemmas that new circumstances and decisions create and resolve them by using facts.

To demonstrate how the implementation of each of the six dimensions works in the real world, I use an example of an integrated system by way of illustration. In this example, a partnership called "NewMed" has maximized all the key concepts of each dimension. A short scenario highlighting their success will be offered at the end of this and each of the next five chapters. These examples draw on the best characteristics of many actual systems around the country that are implementing at least one of the six dimensions. There is a significant difference between NewMed and the real systems that have inspired this book, however. NewMed has mastered all six dimensions at the same time. Although many examples of success in each dimension are described in this book, to date the authors have not found a single system that has maximized the total sequence of critical elements described here.

Readers will probably see similarities to their own system in some of these stories. However, others will sound like the "impossible dream." If the conversations that make up these stories describe your particular situation, you are already leading the transformation to the new practice of medicine. If, however, none of these stories is familiar to your experience, it is time to begin building a strategy to reinvent yourself by seeking out the motivation and innovation described in this book.

A good way to set a strategy for your own practice is to use the concluding examples in Chapters Three through Eight as a barometer. If the story feels impossible, the subject being discussed doesn't represent the right area for early steps. If the example sounds like it could have taken place in your system, but with only half of the issues described actually in place, you have found a good focus for your early agenda for change. Those areas that are already working well will sound familiar within the examples. These areas are strengths. The goal of the new practice is to strengthen all six dimensions until all six of them are working well enough to reinforce each other simultaneously. Leaving any one of the dimensions out completely reduces the overall potential to achieve long-term success. By improving all of them continuously, the new practice of medicine will emerge.

### NewMed Installs Success at a Glance Evidence (SAGE™)

"Hey Kenny, what did your SAGE report show?"

"Income up, of course. How about you?"

"Yea, I'm up, too. It's *painful* to be so good." They both laugh. "We must be one of the top groups in the system."

"Did you see our group's DSM percentage?"

"Yeah! We are at 90 percent implementation of management plans on the pediatric asthma project. Is that good or *what*?" chortled Bob.

"You know what we need to do: Start another improvement project."

"I agree, if we can do asthma with home education and hit 90 percent protocol use in the office, just *think* what we can do with diabetes!"

"Hold on Bob, did you look at the drill down on our report?"

"No, but it's right here."

"Well, look at the results of the practice as a whole compared to your data."

Bob looked at the comparisons and was unimpressed. "The practice as a whole is only at 75 percent implementation and you and I are 96 and 98 percent. I have 75 percent of my patients doing peak flow measurements at home but the practice is only 60 percent. Ninety percent of my patients are on anti-inflammatory meds; the practice is 75 percent. We're trying to reduce the use of theophyllines to 10 percent and the practice is still at 50 percent. My patients are at 20 percent, my emergency room visits are down, my admits are down, but my bonus is based on the practice's success."

Kenny responded, "Well, that's the way it should be."

"Well, if this is justice, I must be missing something."

"Look Bob, our success depends on the group's data. The practice as a whole has to succeed. We need to organize a meeting to help our peers review the data."

Bob and Kenny both looked at the summary report. The "clinical effectiveness" line had a star on it that indicated a statistically significant trend. The incentive bonus was up by $1,201, even though it only represented 65 percent of the maximum achievable bonus.

"Look at this, Kenny. I mean if we are in this together, the rest of the group has to get on board, and you know what that means. There's no reason for all of us not to be at 90 percent on the use of these asthma protocols."

"Well, you know, it's Bill. He's so busy he claims he can't take the time to use the protocols."

"What a joke! The protocol saves time! It decreases the need for visits and adds to our bonus. What do you think it will take to turn the lights on?"

"Well, I say let's only give him part of the bonus until he gets on board."

"That would help everybody. If he can't contribute to the savings, why give him a bonus?"

"Well, it's all about implementation. We just need to get a process in place that helps Bill."

"You are right."

They scanned down their reports to the section on "office effectiveness."

"You know this drill down feature of the interactive reports is really interesting. Unless it's trending up or down, I don't have to waste time going through the data, so I just drill down on areas that have changed. If the SAGE says 'no trend,' I just keep on working."

"How does SAGE do these reports in real time? I saw the report of last month's data on the first week of this month. That's a few days and it's already out. How do they do that?"

"I think it is because SAGE doesn't deal with anything that isn't in the report. SAGE has one goal in life and that is to help us see our success."

They felt satisfied with the plan to educate Bill. Their practices were secure—the report said it all. But there is always room to improve when the motivation is there.

This chapter has introduced the interdependent nature of the six dimensions of the new practice of medicine, with an emphasis on the first and most important reinforcing system: integrated information exchange. Information focused on answering specific questions to guide education and new strategies will remain the common thread from this point forward. Chapter Four builds the argument that the new practice partnerships can find motivation for needed change through aligned incentives.

# 4

# The Second Dimension

## *Aligned Incentives Reward*
## *the Clinical Behavior You Want*

As Chapter Three shows, the power of partnership integration depends on the ability to gather, analyze, and report data. Integrated information exchange, coupled with education across the continuum of care, creates a critical focus for communication in the new practice. Once this dimension is in place, physicians can concentrate on aligning incentives, the focus of this chapter. Physicians often resist change because of the perverse incentives that emerged under the traditional fee-for-service health care system. An old adage states, "You get the behavior you reward." So it goes in health care. New partnerships are rewarding providers who promote good health in addition to high volumes of disease treatment. Patients want to be healthy, yet the health care system of the past did not usually reward good health. By aligning physicians' income with actions that promote patient self-care, decreased disease frequency, and improved medical outcomes, practices can reward themselves for doing more than just providing care.

The second dimension, aligned incentives, builds on the first, integrated information exchange. Without the availability of information across the system, it is difficult to align physicians' economic incentives fairly. Physicians need partnerships that can give them integrated clinical and financial information. The right information and reports can convince physicians that certain changes are safe as well as economically beneficial. This chapter will outline key features of a plan to create incentives for health partners who can prove that the clinical outcomes of care get better as cost is decreased. With this model, physicians and their partners are proving they "do no harm" as they increase their economic success.

## All Care Is Capitated

In general, the payer groups, insurance companies, HMOs, Medicare, Medicaid, and managed care businesses control the cost of purchasing medical care. All of these organizations have a budget that can be viewed as their cap on total revenue. Once this cap is set, they pay providers the real cost of care and accept a loss if they go over budget. HMOs and insurance companies can also keep any profit if they are under budget. All care is delivered under these caps, or ceilings. To create a profit (or in the case of government and nonprofit payers, a financial reserve), the costs of care must be reduced to a point below the cap.

For-profit companies in this third-party-payer system have an obligation to maximize returns to their investors, with little oversight to ensure they are not harming their members. These third-party payers are large enough to take the financial or actuarial risk involved in buying and selling care, thus creating leverage over smaller groups (Halvorson, 1989, p. 110). This ability to leverage power is an important point, since employers usually purchase the vast majority of care from large third-party, for-profit payers. The payer and the employer control reimbursement. Through this exchange of revenue they are able to guide physician reward and shape provider behavior and the services provided. Pneumonia treatment provides an example of how physician behavior is rewarded in traditional or discounted fee-for-service medicine. Under the current system, providers of care get paid more for treating a patient with pneumonia than they would if they used prevention to stave off pneumonia in a given patient (Halvorson, 1989, p. 29).

The new practice of medicine shifts this perverse thinking by putting the provider of care at financial risk for the cost of care. The legal requirements for organizations who accept risk and can therefore share rewards have been tested in many capitated plans across the country. The 1997 Balanced Budget Act was passed to encourage the development of provider-sponsored organizations (PSOs) that act as HMOs. These organizations can be more than 50 percent owned by providers, and they have a three-year deferment on gaining an HMO license. This opportunity will open the door to risk sharing and aligned incentives even further. The common feature of these provider arrangements is that the HMO or PSO fixes reimbursement to the provider, no matter what the cost of care. This model gives the budgeted amount estimated to cover the costs for care to some type of partnership that includes the providers who deliver the care. Providers assume the losses if they overspend, but they can also keep the profit if the real costs of care are below the budget. This is their risk. This method pays the physician more for prevention and effective utilization because the reward is directly linked to physician behavior. For example, an independent practice association (IPA) or physician hospital organization (PHO) working through a managed care organization (MCO) can become at risk by accepting a specific contract to fix the physician reimbursement. If the physician organization then unwisely continues to pay physicians fee-for-service, motivating them to do more, the organization is likely to lose money. This is a concern for those following the success or failure of the recently suggested PSOs. In these provider-sponsored organizations the hospitals and physicians are being lured to take over the third-party responsibilities without investing the time and money to achieve an HMO license for three years. This easy access to full risk contracting encourages new partnerships to jump into the HMO business without a good plan for managing the care. If physicians do not stop doing what they have always been rewarded to do, they will keep providing more care and cause the partnership to go bankrupt.

Many nonprofit HMOs traveled this road as well, trying to keep the physicians happy by paying fee-for-service even though their budget was capped. This circumstance within an integrated system has prevented many health partnerships from succeeding. Physician behavior can bankrupt any plan that starts taking on risk while rewarding higher volumes of care. Unfortunately, this mismatch between incentives and behavior is often ignored until it leads to financial failure.

## Watching the Flow of Money

Physicians need to be inspired in order to include new preventive and high-efficiency behavior in their practice. The best way to persuade physicians is to show them who gets what portion of the health care dollars when physicians change clinical care. Every dollar the patient, the employer, or the government pays for care is allocated to some part of the delivery system to cover health care expenses. With a basic understanding of how third-party payers are organized and a few simple calculations, physicians can see an estimate of who gets how much money (Solomon, 1997, pp. 132–140).

The best way to analyze reward is to examine how the premium dollar is split between the groups that make up the delivery system. This distribution of revenue changes when the physicians are paid under different contracts. Under each type of reimbursement model, income either goes up or down based on volume, quality of care, and an agreed-upon split of the premium dollar.

Seeing the financial impact of improvement strategies under different contracts is critical for success. When the physician is paid more or less in the current system, some other part of the delivery system is also seeing a change in its portion of the premium dollar. With this information clarified, physicians can evaluate fair and unfair situations. The new partnerships must have a strong commitment to communication and to fairness at this point or else conflict will ensue. If one part of the new interdependent partnership improves its financial opportunity, it could decrease the opportunity for another part of the partnership. This situation, in turn, will create resentment. Education and a plan for achieving fairness must immediately be put in place. If this feeling of disparity is ignored after the circumstance is exposed, and no commitment to fairness exists, it can create all-out war. The goals of the new partnerships are to support the achievement of visible fairness through accurate measurement, education, motivated new behavior, and success for all. Otherwise, information can cause more harm than good.

## Seeing the Difference Between the Budget and the Cost

Physicians need to keep in mind that all care is provided under a cap. Figure 4.1 illustrates two ways to divide up the profit if the health care providers spend less on care than their cap or budget. In this example, the first set of figures outlines the payer's plan to split up the premium dollar. Twenty percent is budgeted to the insurance company. Forty percent is budgeted to cover hospital costs, and forty percent to cover the physician costs. To create a profit, the payer attempts to come in below the 20 percent budgeted for operations. But the potential profit is much greater if provider costs are lowered below the budgeted 80 percent. In a profitable year, the amount of money the insurance companies spend on patient care is less than the amount collected from their members. Because payers accept the risk of losses if they go over budget, they are also entitled to the difference when their costs are lower than the cap. That is where the profit comes from in the insurance business.

The insurance companies' profit or loss is based on how much they collect from policyholders, less what they spend on care and their own overhead. To calculate the payer's profit, one must total the insurance reimbursement portion of the hospital and physician revenue. This includes pharmacy, home health, and ancillary services. This amount is then subtracted from their total revenue. For

**Figure 4.1. Why Align Incentives?**

Distribution Choices/Splitting the Premium Dollar

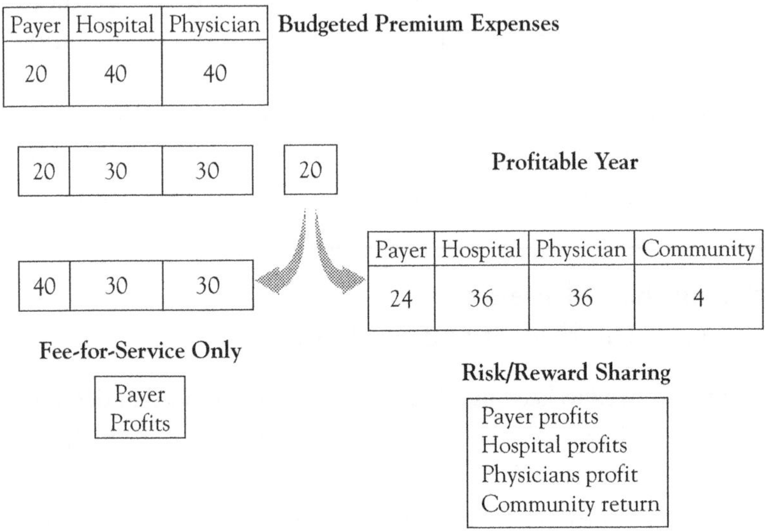

| Payer | Hospital | Physician |
|-------|----------|-----------|
| 20 | 40 | 40 |

Budgeted Premium Expenses

| | | |
|---|---|---|
| 20 | 30 | 30 |

| |
|---|
| 20 |

**Profitable Year**

| Payer | Hospital | Physician | Community |
|-------|----------|-----------|-----------|
| 24 | 36 | 36 | 4 |

| | | |
|---|---|---|
| 40 | 30 | 30 |

**Fee-for-Service Only**

| Payer Profits |
|---|

**Risk/Reward Sharing**

| Payer profits |
|---|
| Hospital profits |
| Physicians profit |
| Community return |

instance, in a good year for the payer, the actual cost of purchasing the provider's care declines because of the hospital's and the physician's efficiency. As a result of their efficiency, the provider actually receives less money whereas the insurance company profits. The left-hand column in Figure 4.1 shows how this works.

A portion of the corporate profit could be used to reward providers for their efficiency if payers wanted to share corporate profits with hospitals, physicians, and the community. Rather than distributing profit to stockholders, these companies could improve the health of their patients, achieve better outcomes, and add efficiency to care by rewarding providers for these outcomes.

If, however, prevention is not reinforced with some type of reward, physicians will not begin disease management and prevention programs quickly and those that are started will not be sustained. Rewarding physicians who create savings with better and more efficient care is an example of a reinforcing loop. By withdrawing savings that physicians and hospitals are creating, payers bring this reinforcing loop to a dead stop.

The ethics behind typical payer arrangements are highly questionable. When a for-profit business needs to cut its losses to make a profit, it is likely to do so. With a legal obligation to maximize profit, the CEOs of insurance companies could consider overt rationing of care to overcome declining reimbursement. If everyone would apply systems thinking to this situation, communities and physicians could not fail to see the catastrophic consequences of continuing on the current course.

The short-term profits that can be achieved by cutbacks have lured an entire industry away from professional accountability, and patients are the most likely to suffer in the end. Insurance companies are businesses motivated by Wall Street investors who demand that profits be used for acquisition or converted to quarterly dividends and distributed to stockholders. The new practice of medicine is more concerned with the health of the community than with investor dividends, but to have an impact these new health partnerships will have to learn the principles of third-party payment. Physicians and hospitals must build partnerships that prove they can manage the care well enough to be competitive. At that point, the new partnerships can build negotiation leverage with the payers.

A good example of this philosophy will evolve out of what is likely to be the first provider-sponsored organization, or PSO, in the country. St. Joseph's Health Care in Albuquerque, New Mexico, has started this ball rolling first because of the flexibility of the New Mexico state insurance commission. Some prominent physicians who will be partners in this PSO are leading the effort with St. Joseph's to improve the care to the elderly. They feel that this PSO as a competitive insurance product has the potential to sweep the state for one reason: The physicians will drive it. They are even willing to lose money until St. Joseph's gets the critical number of patients to succeed.

The model described by the lower right-hand column of Figure 4.1 represents this type of new practice strategy, whether it evolves in partnership with a for-profit HMO or a not-for-profit provider-sponsored organization. No matter which organization plugs into the payer box, this model has a number of advantages. It rewards the physician, hospital, and community when the cooperative effort has proven to help decrease health care costs by improving health. This fair redistribution of revenues can be used to motivate providers and the community. Because it can actually motivate those who provide care to achieve better health for their patients, this model contains immense potential for the new practice of medicine.

Not-for-profit HMOs in the Minneapolis, St. Paul area are also implementing this model. These HMOs are partnering with physicians under strategies that share profits when health statistics improve. Several health indicators have shown steady improvement, including the frequency of myocardial infarction. This is a result of prevention added to the care strategy.

## Calculating Savings and Incentivizing Behavior in the Transition

The majority of physicians will need to restructure their work and rewards under the new practice of medicine by working in both the fee-for-service world and the capitated or shared-risk contracting world, especially where Medicare and Medicaid HMO products are being offered.

It is important to understand simple financial principles. There will always be a set amount of money that will be used to cover the cost of care. It will be distributed in at least one of three predominant models: the for-profit fee-for-service insurance model, the HMO model offering sub caps, or the new practice of medicine model sharing full risk. Most practices will have a mixture of all three.

## Fee-for-Service (FFS)

The for-profit insurance model rewards the physician under discounted FFS, which increases revenue only if the amount of care provided increases. Physicians are signing these contracts out of fear of losing patient volume. Even with discounts whereby the third party pays the physician less per unit of care, the overall cost of providing care to the community could continue to increase if the volume of procedures and treatments goes up to keep the physicians' incomes stable. To track the money in this model it is necessary to find out what amount the insurance company uses to calculate what they are willing to pay out on a per-member per-month (pm pm) basis. This amount is available from the insurance company at the time of contracting, although most physicians see no point in asking what it is. This amount usually ranges from $70 to $200 (pm pm).

The insurance company usually budgets between 20 and 30 percent of the gross revenue to advertise, handle the money, process bills, and of course profit. The remainder of their real cost is the amount paid out.

To see an estimate of the payer's profit it is necessary to subtract their costs from the actual revenue that they generate. The insurance company's revenue is calculated by taking the members' premium amount, multiplied by the total membership under the payer's contracts. The real costs can only be calculated by totaling what is paid to the providers, including lab and pharmacy. The costs are easy to calculate from a conceptual perspective, but because there have been no incentives to look, most providers have seldom seen where the real profits in the system could be shared.

Because costs go up as more total money is paid out for more care being delivered, the insurer can create economic success by pressuring providers to limit care. Pre-authorization and pharmacy formularies that limit care options are a common strategy to achieve this success. The insurance carrier can also contract with providers to get them to accept discounts per unit of care. The problem for the third-party payer is that this FFS model doesn't ensure profit. Because this model still rewards more patient volume per provider, as the revenue per visit drops, the need for more patient visits per provider emerges as a strategy to maintain income. That also means less physician time must be spent per person seen unless a lower cost provider such as a physician's assistant is used to see the patient.

This model doesn't incentivize physicians to provide better care even though it motivates them to see more patients. Another long-term problem for these physicians as a whole is that this shift in motivation actually lowers the need for physicians. Eventually a physician in this model must drop whatever care is too time consuming and not reimbursed. This scenario is the one that is most familiar to the majority of physicians in America. Too many physicians are asking insurance carriers to slow the rate that they are decreasing discounts and calling that a success. This so-called success eliminates the hope for fair incentives and eventually pushes physicians to ration the time spent with patients, while they continue to compete with each other, all of which helps the payer maintain control.

### Calculating the Impact of Contracts

Most practicing physicians are paying themselves in FFS production models even if they are in large groups accepting HMO-type contracts that place them at risk under a cap. For these physicians to make informed decisions about their future, they must be able to calculate the financial impact that occurs when they create changes in clinical volume and type of care. This requires measuring revenue from the payer and calculating the expenses incurred during the care. The next step is to apply the calculations to each insurance plan in which they participate. This type of business thinking is called cost-volume-profit (CVP) analysis.

To gain understanding of profit, physicians can estimate the hourly wage they make under each contract as they provide improvements in care that affect cost and volume. These calculations can be done several ways. The most basic way is to take the total costs and subtract that amount from the total collections, which are then divided by the number of hours that the physician works.

$$\text{(Total collections} - \text{total cost)/} \\ \text{(No. of hours worked)} = \text{Hourly wage}$$

This gives an overall average hourly wage.

The physician can also take the number of patients seen in a given week and divide that number by the number of hours worked. This gives a patient seen per hour average.

$$\text{(No. of patients seen per week)/(No. of hours worked} \\ \text{per week)} = \text{Average no. of patients seen per hour}$$

Another method to add detail is to ask the front desk to track the number of patients seen per hour by reviewing the office ledger. The percentage of total patients seen by payer contract can also be calculated from simply sorting the bills by contract. This number can then be used to calculate what percentage of the fixed overhead should be applied against the money collected in each contract. This calculation is a reasonable estimate of the profit by contract, which can easily be broken down into hourly wage.

When the amount of total cost including fixed overhead is subtracted from the collections by contract, that number can be divided by the number of patients. This gives profit per patient by contract.

$$\text{(Collections} - \text{expense for specific patient care} \\ \text{under contract A)/(No. of patients with A as payer)} = \\ \text{Profit per patient under contract A}$$

By multiplying this number (profit per patient) by the number of patients seen per hour, a contract-specific hourly wage emerges.

When physicians calculate collections less expense by contract and see the hourly wage, bad contracts begin to show themselves. Most physicians are startled by doing this calculation for each payer contract because of the varying levels of hourly wage that are already in place.

Reducing physician cost remains the goal of most payers. From their perspective, deeper discounted FFS has paid off, leaving physicians with the problem of finding a way to maintain their income. Surprisingly, few physicians have a plan to do anything about this payer strategy.

## Sub-Capitation Shifts the Risk to the Providers

As managed care becomes more widespread, some payers will offer to place the physician at risk for economic losses through giving them a sub-cap. This occurs when the payer estimates the cost as a set dollar amount that will guarantee them a profit. They then attempt to get the providers to accept this amount as a contract, giving them the risk of going over this amount. This is what most physicians think of as a capitated contract. It eliminates the payer's risk and adds little to ensure the success of the provider.

The HMO in this case, like all payers, handles the money as it is collected from its members. The HMO then pays out its budgeted dollars to the providers on a fixed schedule regardless of patient volume. Unlike FFS, the contracted providers get to keep more money if they provided less care. The HMO gets a guaranteed profit, which is the difference between the collections they get from members of their plan and the physician's capped payment. The problem with this model is that in the past it has been implemented without sufficient monitoring of clinical data. In this old HMO model, rationing could occur in a variety of ways and no one would actually see it. Providers could remove the expensive, high-tech specialty care by using gatekeepers. They could limit expensive drugs or tests and no one would know unless a serious complication occurred. Even in cases of injury, less than one in ten would go to a lawsuit, and most of these would be won by the providers (Brennan, 1991, pp. 370–376).

To track the financial success of this model, the physicians have to measure their real practice costs. They can then allocate a percentage of these costs to each contract based on patient volume as described above. By subtracting the appropriate portion of overhead based on volume from each capitated contract payment, a profit or loss can be demonstrated. Next, the number of patient visits seen under each payer contract is used to divide the total payment into a per patient amount. This allows a calculation of what the physician actually gets paid for a single patient. It is then possible to take the number of patients usually seen per hour, and multiply the amount made per patient times this number. This gives an hourly wage for each capitated plan that can be compared to the other plans.

**Cap payment in contract = Gross contract specific income**

**Gross contract specific income – Portion of overhead based on patients seen = Profit under contract**

**(Profit under contract)/(No. of visits) = Net income under contract per visit**

**Net income per visit × Visits per hour = Hourly wage by contract**

It is sound business thinking to see the difference in actual hourly wage paid for these capitated plans, just as it is under FFS. It is this amount, tracked as increasing or decreasing wage, that defines the economic value of one contract over another.

For example, an office practice income for a three-physician practice could be $800,000. Fifteen percent of the $800,000 could also be under capitation, or $120,000. The overhead before salary is 50 percent ($400,000). The physicians have 5,000 patient encounters each or 15,000 total. By patient count, they had 1,500 encounters with capitated patients. It is reasonable to assume that each physician would have about 500 patients visits each.

The practice allocates 10 percent of the total overhead to correspond to the patient volume (1,500 of 15,000 encounters). Overhead for capitated patients is $400,000 multiplied by 10 percent, which equals $40,000. The calculation to reach net income per patient is capped income ($120,000) minus overhead ($40,000), which equals ($80,000). This amount is then divided by 1,500, which equals $53.34 per patient.

**(Capped income [$120,000] – Overhead [$40,000] = $80,000)/(1,500 Capitated patients) = $53.34 per patient**

If the physicians can see 5 patients per hour, then hourly wage is $266 per hour, and each physician earns $53.34 multiplied by 500 encounters or $26,600 out of this patient population. This amount is what is earned for seeing only 10 percent of the total patient volume.

In another circumstance, in the same contract year they could have earned the same income of $800,000 with the same $120,000 under a capped contract and the same 50 percent overhead. This time let's say they only have 4,000 encounters each per year for a total of 12,000, and the capitated patient visit count goes up to 3,000 encounters or about 1000 for each physician. In this circumstance, the percentage overhead for capitated patients will go up to 25 percent of the total corresponding to the 3,000 out of 12,000 encounters, yet the income will be fixed.

Twenty-five percent of the $400,000 overhead is $100,000. The calculation is now $120,000 (capped income) minus $100,000 (overhead) equals $20,000 (profit) divided by 3,000 (number of visits). This equals $6.67 per patient in this population.

**(Capped income [$120,000] – Overhead [$100,000] = $20,000)/3,000 Capitated patients = $6.67 per patient**

That means that if a physician can only see 4 patients per hour, their hourly wage is $26.68 per hour, and each physician earns approximately 1,000 times 6.67 or $6,670 for the capitated patient population.

It is easy to see that lower productivity and unnecessarily high patient encounters work against the practice and physician income under this type of a contract.

HMOs can profit by shifting the risk to physicians through a sub-cap; they also lower the need for physicians. Because primary care profit can come from less specialty care being provided, specialists are sparingly used. The "gatekeeper" model was developed by HMOs to keep patients under the care of primary care physicians whenever possible. Little research has been conducted to measure the clinical impact of this model, in part because HMOs have not set aside enough money for such studies. As a result, the long-term effects of this model are unknown. The failure to treat, diagnose, or refer to a specialist has led to a growing number of lawsuits. In particular, California has experienced a significant increase in lawsuits against family practitioners in the past several years (Richards and others, 1997, pp. 443–473).

One of the major flaws with this system is that physicians profited by withholding care regardless of clinical impact. In addition, HMOs guaranteed a profit for themselves by shifting the risk of economic losses to the provider. This strategy had another major flaw—the physicians were not trained in a delivery method that gave them the opportunity for financial success. Because of these flaws, most physicians believe that managed care is not the solution.

### The New Practice Model

The new practice of medicine strives to do what is right for the patient, the provider, and the community. Corruption or neglect is possible in any system, but the new practice model has several unique checks and balances. Decreases in overall health care costs are justified by clinical data (facts) and a professional commitment to improve care through disease state management. That is much different from the traditional HMO model because there are new costs that must be taken into account. For example, the new practice model requires education and setting up a technical measurement infrastructure, which becomes an investment in patient care. Patients are involved in saving money for the provider. This situation motivates physicians to take on the expense to educate their patients and implement efficient prevention services.

The community partners who participate in the new practice, such as businesses or public health, can also have access to the summary of clinical and cost data, including the flow of money relating to cost of illness and improvements in care. In this collaborative effort, the health system acts more like a physician hospital community organization (PHCO) than what we have come to think of as an HMO. These cooperative organizations, like the one formed recently in Spokane, Washington, are a partnership with businesses, hospitals, and physicians. Together, they decide how to use some of the savings to fund more health promotion in the community rather than just distributing the profit to stockholders. Physicians and hospitals are motivated to improve quality, efficiency, prevention, and sustained recovery because all of these strategies not only benefit the community, but also create personal economic reward.

This cooperative organization (or PHCO) controls the premium dollar and uses 10 to 24 percent to cover third-party administration cost and to stockpile reserves for reinvestment. As with insurance companies and HMOs, the PHCO sets a cap on dollars that it budgets to pay for providers' care. But providers who save money by providing less care are obligated to show that disease management data also demonstrate access, satisfaction, and better clinical outcomes.

Best care creates a profit for the providers and the community as the PHCO grows because there is an agreement from all parties to retain some of the PHCO savings for the community. Unfortunately, the new practice model also lowers the need for physicians because it relies more on allied health and nursing personnel, home health educators, and quality improvement managers to provide education and care. But this approach does contain a number of positive features. By decreasing the need for disease treatment, reducing the overall cost of care, and documenting improved community health, the new practice model has a much more predictable impact on the future of health care. In addition, the physicians using this model have the added reassurance that the highest professional standards are being maintained as well as their own job security.

*Calculating the Benefits of Disease State Management*

Physicians will see that they can get paid a higher hourly wage under PHCO contracts for aggressive disease management than either FFS or capitated contracts. Because the quality of clinical care is measured and best care is more cost effective, the physician can be properly rewarded when care improves. The PHCO system is more fair from the physician's perspective. The example of pneumonia management made this point clear earlier. All would agree that the faster the patient recovers and the less often patients get pneumonia, the better.

To begin in the new practice, providers must calculate the savings and losses within each of their contracts to determine visible fairness in the delivery of care to these patients. The physicians in a practice need to take this information and decide through face-to-face dialogue what they will consider to be visible fairness. Finally, they must resolve whether they want to change their approach based on an accounting of facts.

*The New Practice of Medicine*

Assumption of risk forces the new practices to take the time for prevention or lose the revenue that is spent on acute care. The simple intervention for pneumonia shown in Figure 4.2 can create significant savings and a bonus through aligned incentives. In Minneapolis St. Paul, a medical group established the addition of volunteers, called "naggers," who were willing to call elderly patients daily to get flu shots. By increasing the frequency of flu shots

**Figure 4.2. The New Practice Strategy Pays Off in Capitation.**

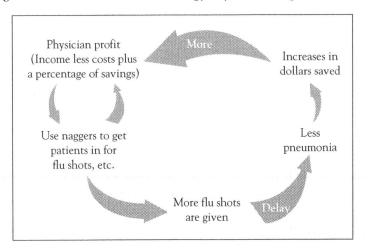

they reduced hospitalizations for pneumonia in their patients. This simple success created a savings from the real cost of care and the projected cost. This scenario works only if physician practices are provided with incentives to partner with both the hospital and the community to strategize and plan for improvement.

The goal of the new practice of medicine is to save the patient from illness wherever disease management research has proven that it is possible. New practices invest in the cost of prevention and achieve a return on that investment. This investment is not without risk, of course. The real costs of patient care, plus education and prevention, are subtracted from the fixed revenue allocated to cover the cost of care of this population. The provider's revenue then increases in an agreed upon formula if less care is needed. The improvement is clearly illustrated in Figure 4.2.

In contrast to the old models, with their perverse incentives, the new practice of medicine highlights the benefit of aligning economic reward with long-term disease management and illness prevention.

## Critical Elements for Aligning Incentives

- Access to financial and clinical data is linked to contracts for reimbursement.

- The contracts spell out risk sharing or the lack of it.

- Financial forecasting is done as an accounting method.

- The cost, volume, and profit are accounted for in order to see the amount available for reward after expenses.

- Calculations of hourly physician wage are made for each payer contract.

- Payers willing to share full risk or put a ceiling on potential profits are sought out as partners.

- Physician, hospital, and community partnerships are formed that make managing the diseases of a population profitable under a fixed budget.

- Disease state management and demand management strategies are implemented.

- Physician skills in dialogue, conflict resolution, and negotiation regarding disease state management are developed.

### NewMed Begins to Implement Aligned Incentives

The business meetings had taken on a new importance since the group had decided to accept shared-risk contracts. Although the HMO that the NewMed Health System was trying to support had started out slowly, it was clearly becoming the favorite contract of the group practices.

"This won't take long." Kenny turned on the LCD panel projector to display the summary report.

Bill's skepticism was visible, "Does this really have last month's data in it?"

"It certainly does." Kenny said, "This table adds the most recent month's data within a week of the data collection, and updates the trend chart."

"Let's start with the dollars. The raw figures aren't as important as the trends."

"You can see that the overall revenue is increasing a little," Bill added.

"I know our participation in disease state management is higher than everybody else's. We actually do manage the patient, rather than the disease. We've got home education going on—just look at our percentage on protocols for asthma. Why aren't we making more money?"

Kenny showed the drill down report for the asthma. At a glance, it was clear that this "practice accountable for quality" (PAQ) was well above average compared to other groups.

Kenny paged back to the cover report and drilled down on the cost-effectiveness data. "This report includes a breakdown of all the important figures. The overall bonus from DSM only applies to the NewMed contract. It is up, but it only represented 10 percent of the patients."

Bob added, "The other fee-for-service contracts didn't reward the practice, and it is clear that fee-for-service revenue was not increased even though the implementation of protocols and frequency of admits shows clear success for the management of disease."

Kenny drilled down on profit by individual contracts. "The bonuses for the NewMed HMO are high enough that the practice was actually getting more money per patient for these encounters than in the old days."

Kenny interrupted, "The discounted FFS contracts are another story. They not only show a zero in the bonus column, but the reimbursement per patient is 30 percent lower than full fees and 50 percent lower than the NewMed patients."

"The hourly wage figures say it all." Broken down by contract, the figures were clearly irritating to the group.

"Well it's right here, Bill. The lowest reimbursing plans represent 10 percent of the patient volume, but only 7 percent of the revenue." They paused.

Kenny was the first to break the silence. "Well, are we busy enough to drop those contracts?" There was another long pause.

Bob's eyes scanned the reports. "I see the logic in that Kenny. It would increase our overall hourly wage if we can fill the patient openings with new patients. How do we know that is possible?"

"Well, that's easy to figure," Bill said. "How many of us have a wait time for new patient appointments? Kenny, do you even take new patients?"

"Not really, but I could fill the spaces if I had any, especially if it makes sense for the practice."

"We still have a diversity of contracts, so we are safe," Bill reemphasized. "We are just making room for those patients who can improve our hourly wage."

This chapter has outlined the essential principles and steps needed to create clear motivation through aligned incentives. However, some physicians will remain skeptical and unclear on whether or not they should take financial risk, even if rewards are demonstrated through clear regular reports. Physician change is difficult—as it should be. Physicians should not agree to these strategies until they are confident that decreasing the volume of care will not harm the practice.

Chapter Five outlines the third, and possibly the most important, dimension of the transformation toward a new practice of medicine. It focuses on techniques of clinical process improvement, evidence-based medicine, and disease state management as techniques to change clinical care. The support needed to put these techniques in place makes it possible for physicians to lead the transformation.

# 5

# The Third Dimension
## *Improving the Process of Care and the Clinical Outcome with CPI*

The last two chapters clarified the potential to track and report success in order to reward the new partnerships. Once these two dimensions are in place, the structure exists to support a continuous improvement of clinical care. Some organizations have been unable to implement clinical process improvement (CPI) even though the systems thinking and the integrated information necessary for such a change have been in place for several years. This chapter focuses on overcoming the barriers to CPI.

Getting the best outcome at the lowest cost is a critical success factor for the new practice of medicine. In addition to economic success the goal is to show an impact on the health of the population as a whole.

CPI (adapted from the managerial philosophy of total quality management/continuous quality improvement [TQM/CQI]) has been taught as a method for improving medical care for nearly ten years. As experience with CPI grows, clinical outcomes and research on disease state management are providing a growing body of medical literature (Berwick, 1998). Landmark texts and recent additions to the literature are included in the Recommended Reading section at the end of this book to expand the reader's understanding of specific improvement methods. Physician leaders in this effort included Brent James, Donald Berwick, Paul Bataldin, David Blumenthal, Lucian Leape, and recently many others. All of the CPI efforts directed by these individuals and their organizations are dedicated to clinical process change and improved outcomes. To succeed, physicians need information, because CPI follows the principles of large, population-based, historically controlled, nonrandomized, nonblinded clinical trials (James, 1989, p. 34). The results of individual care are collected and then grouped to describe the real care that has occurred in one year compared to the year before. This research is similar to that done for cancer drugs without the clinical controls, randomization, or blinding techniques. Because it is not a scientifically robust design, it can't be used for investigation. However, outcomes research has the advantage of much smaller populations without the burden of the rigorous research methods required for investigation. Outcomes improvement focuses on one diagnosis at a time, so the research requirements are simple enough to be managed by a quality improvement professional on a personal computer.

This body of knowledge has now spread worldwide through education, information sharing, and networks such as the Health Care Forum, Institute for Healthcare Improvement (IHI), the VHA, Inc., the Veteran's Administration (VA), and the American Hospital Association (AHA). A quick glance at the reading list shows that many dedicated individual practices and hospitals have become experts in improving care and sharing the lessons learned. Intermountain Health Care (IHC) has proven that in some diagnoses such as adult respiratory distress syndrome and postoperative wound infection, medical outcomes can be improved four- and five-fold over the national average (Morris and others, 1994, pp. 295–305). These dramatic successes are accomplished through a clear, well-planned series of steps that measure the variation in care and replace what doesn't work with what does. The real challenge is to encourage a decrease in variation and move toward consistent best practice. This step requires physicians to change how they make medical decisions. Once that step is accomplished, the results are simply measured.

There are several ways to measure and report the change in approaches to clinical care. In many cases these approaches can be defined by explicit process criteria linked to associated outcomes. All of these approaches equate to what is now called *clinical quality.*

It is possible to assess the frequency of error-free delivery of a given clinical criterion applied to a population of patients. It is also possible to look at all of the care given to a single patient, focusing on the percentage of recommended process steps taken. In the latter case, physicians assess how many steps within a pathway are accomplished in order to calculate the proportion of the total possible steps as a type of implementation success rate. Steps that are omitted can also be taken as a percentage, which gives an error rate. The percentage of physicians achieving the goal to use a specific protocol criteria is another way to look at the success of implementing change across a group of physicians. The percentage of goals achieved can be summarized in every component of the new partnerships and reports can be used to show overall system success. The percentage of improvement goals achieved can be measured for a system of any size. All of these methods create meaningful measures of the new practice partnership's success or lack thereof in improving quality.

By clearly outlining best-practice process steps at the outset, the proportion of steps that are met defines the success or depth of groupwide adoption of best practice. This success directly affects the cost of care and the bill for services in a fee-for-service world. This powerful approach can help a great deal with financial forecasting. When process steps and a specific outcome are known to be associated, physicians can predict improvement in the outcome by simply implementing the process step. As explained in the last chapter, the decrease in cost can be calculated with simple cost-volume-profit analysis.

After a proportion of process steps have been adopted and consistently put in place, physicians using CPI can predict which outcomes will improve. This clinical-financial forecast creates a target goal. Once that goal is achieved, it will begin to create rewards.

Any type of care without explicit process criteria or a defined, agreed-upon standard should not be a part of this strategy. This type of care is simply too difficult to analyze. Any medical decision that is not black and white is inappropriate for building incentives for improvement. This type of care can only be evaluated subjectively by using the best judgment of a group of committed and accomplished professionals. The new practice partnerships realize this and determine which of these gray areas of care are usual and customary and therefore adequate.

Experts can also suggest areas of care that may have room for improvement, but this is a purely subjective decision. Efficiency and the intention to use good clinical judgment are the only strategies that can be applied in these situations.

## Knowing What to Change

When choosing a CPI candidate, remember that the more subjective the outcome being evaluated, the less reliable the analysis is statistically. Any unreliable outcome should not be used to direct change or reward. Patient satisfaction, understanding of instructions, involvement in the decision, and informed consent are important but do not usually lend themselves to CPI analysis.

More suitable areas for CPI are found within the many guidelines and quality of care criteria that are now more widely published as disease state management (DSM) or evidence-based medicine (EBM) (Siegel, 1998, p. 1395). DSM and EBM are simple research approaches, in contrast to the randomized controlled trials and multivariable observational studies applied to expert opinion. The Institute of Medicine and the Agency for Health Care Policy and Research have popularized these complex approaches (Blumenthal and Scheck, 1995).

The randomized controlled trial process is extremely important but it is so complex and expensive that it has been unable to show a widespread impact on actual clinical practice outcomes. This process is difficult to implement and often lacks the statistical significance that can be achieved with single variable CPI studies. In addition, data collection is burdensome. Because the impact of each of the process variables often cannot be adequately adjusted for, this complex approach has not proven to be usable as a research tool for practicing physicians. Providers of care in actual practice need a practical tool and the support to use it. Because CPI focuses on individual steps proven to make a difference through outcomes, research, and evidence-based protocols, it is a good starting point for change.

## Thinking in Terms of CPI

With CPI, physicians have a real opportunity to be rewarded for contributing to best care through consistent, error-free implementation of the explicit process steps proven in the literature to affect outcomes. Simple guidelines, rapid feedback on performance, and specific education by peers are all that physicians need to implement the chosen process steps successfully. This approach will lead to measurably improved care, but only if the physicians' organization guides physicians to the appropriate process steps and supports them in their effort to change.

CPI theory states that if genuine new advances come from the investigational literature, and good research clarifies the value of a new process step, this step can become a candidate for CPI. If physicians identify a process step in the literature that will improve outcomes if implemented, it would seem that they would simply need to follow CPI protocol to improve results in care. Those who have succeeded with CPI models know, however, that it takes more than theory to keep specific process steps in place. The new partnerships are using the CPI model not only to change the outcomes of patient care but also to influence physician behavior.

Drawing heavily on common sense and reward, this model of research can improve actual clinical practice. Simply stated, CPI points the way to those clinical process steps that, if taken consistently and on time, improve the delivery of care. Chapter Six will describe how high performance and new physician behavior can be achieved, but first physicians in a practice must agree that CPI theory is legitimate and that change is safe.

## Doing a Feasibility Analysis for CPI

An effective way to begin implementing CPI strategies is to build a financial and implementation plan to guide and motivate an improvement effort. If the plan cannot be described on paper, it will certainly fail. The following plan was developed by Medical Resource Management (MRM) as a modification of the Intermountain Health Care (IHC) approach to CPI (Prather, 1998, p. 111). The plan has been expanded to include steps in data management that are not automated in most systems. It is designed to help organizations expand their understanding of the feasibility of CPI projects before they risk a false start. It organizes and simplifies the principles of CPI implementation and financial forecasting. The only support needed for this simple plan is a PC. However, physicians often will not engage at this early stage of detail. These steps must be done by quality support personnel until physicians realize it is not a waste of their time to do this kind of legwork.

### Step One: Build the Opportunity Statement

The first step in determining feasibility is to describe the opportunity for improvement and savings in detail. This process is similar to the first step taken in an actual CPI project. The opportunity statement contains information pertaining to eleven questions outlined on the next few pages. Quality improvement decision makers must commit to all of the following steps on paper if physicians are to support the project. If the improvement project is described as a clear opportunity, it is much more likely to succeed.

1. *Why is this opportunity important?* Begin with a simple title such as "Reducing Postoperative Wound Infection." Next, ask whether the providers can reduce this complication to a specific point. For instance, if postoperative wound infections can be reduced to one-half of the current rate, from 3 percent to 1.5 percent, the partnership will save at least $200,000 a year in care. This figure was arrived at because it is the amount not reimbursed by Medicare or global HMO contracts for complications. Another important point to emphasize is the impact this change will have on patients. For instance, in this example preventing postoperative wound infection would save lives. Taken together, this is clearly an important opportunity.

2. *What is the clinical volume?* Next, list the number of patients eligible to be studied. In our example, the practice estimates 3,500 surgical cases per year. A set number of these would be clean or clean-contaminated cases that may benefit from prophylactic antibiotics.

3. *How important is it?* Define the clinical importance of the opportunity. In this example the clinical importance could be defined as follows: "Our infections rate is about average, but we know of other systems that have a four times lower infection rate by using prophylactic antibiotics given two hours prior to surgery in the majority (96 percent) of eligible patients." Define it clearly and specifically.

4. *What is the financial impact?* Outline what portion of the patients are in each type of contract. Under Medicare and some managed care, complications may not be covered, so prevention of the complication creates a savings. But care under fee-for-service (FFS) reimbursement needs to be subtracted from the above profits because it pays physicians to manage the complications. Shared-risk contracts open the door to shared savings when care speeds recovery, stops complications, or prevents illness. However, until all care is at shared-risk, the FFS losses must be accounted for.

5. *What is the relationship of this project to previous work?* The opportunity statement should state how this opportunity relates to present and past projects. For instance the present project may benefit from building computerized links among lab, pharmacy, and scheduling. The project might tie into TQM or CQI programs that have been established by management as part of an effort to make these quality teams more clinical in focus. A CPI project may also educate physicians in the understanding of shared risk.

6. *Where will the data come from?* Going through this thought process of a CPI project forces the leaders of the health care partnership to address the location and accessibility of data. To implement most projects some new data collection will be required. It is important to be specific as to the needs in the report. For example, the time of drug dose administration in the operating room (OR) may not be currently entered into a database.

7. *Who will be the physician champion?* A physician champion describes the project to peers and confirms that the data are credible. Always look for a physician champion prior to setting up a project. A respected physician's personal commitment to change is all some projects require.

8. *Who will be on the CPI team?* If the above steps can be accomplished, the next challenge is to define and recruit a CPI team consisting of individuals who are capable of designing and conducting the research. Start by listing individuals who are committed to CPI and the new practice of medicine. Some of these individuals might include quality improvement experts, human resource experts, and individuals with the fundamental knowledge to redesign clinical care. Nurses and physicians are also critical members of the team. It is a good idea to seek commitment from members of the team to stay together and spearhead each and every phase of the CPI process. A team leader is often needed to assume the responsibility of implementation.

9. *What is the rationale?* Next, start your rationale statement by asking why this improvement is possible. In our example, the pre-

vention of postoperative wound infection is related to having peak serum levels of the antibiotic when the incision is made. Although this practice is widely accepted as a concept of best care, antibiotics are given too soon or too late over 50 percent of the time. If the drug is administered properly and consistently, the literature confirms that a portion of these infections can be prevented regardless of the choice of antibiotic (James, and others, 1994, p. 39).

10. *What is the link between process and outcomes?* The report should include a statement of how the link between process and outcome will be documented. For example, the team may want to state the specific thesis that if the drug is given on time, the complication of postoperative deep wound infection for clean-contaminated cases will decrease. In turn, this will change the need for *recovery therapy*, defined as all care needed to return the patient to a state of sustained recovery from the original complication. Include a list of cited references in this section.

11. *What are the measurement indicators?* Describe the key measurement indicators of process and outcome and clarify specific pieces of information that will define success. In our example this would include positive cultures in pathology, a check-off list for signs and symptoms of infection, drug administration data, the time and frequency of doses, and the condition of the patient at the two-week postoperative visit. Unit-based costs of the drug and steps in care are also important to include. In our example, the complications being prevented on occasion include sepsis and even ICU admissions. Therefore, calculate a baseline on cost of caring for all patients with complications being prevented by the study. The new data will be compared to the baseline to show improvement, so only those indicators that will be used in these comparisons need to be included.

### Step Two: Build the Work Plan

To proceed to step two, the planners need to describe the major steps needed to carry out the improvement project in a specific and simple way. For instance, the team might ask, "Who will give the drug?" Possible answers might include the nurse, pharmacist, anesthesiologist, surgeon, or other physician. The team will need to decide where the relevant data will be collected, entered, analyzed, and applied. They will determine the responsible individuals for each step who will also present the results. If the project is to succeed, there must be a specific individual responsible for the results. These specific individuals and their commitment to change will enable the organization to achieve accountability for implementation.

*Timeline.* Place the steps into a written timeline along with the task and responsible party's name.

*Test implementation.* Describe the major steps it will take to test the implementation of the project. With wound infection, the usual method of running the OR, pharmacy, intake, and postoperative floors will guide the step-wise plan. When data are collected, list responsible individuals by name and outline the methods they will use to achieve their tasks by a specific date. Putting this sequence in writing will help to make it a reality.

*Analysis.* Decide what major steps are required to analyze results. Keep it simple and stick to basic chi-squared analysis that can be done with off-the-shelf software packages. Limit the analysis plan to one central process at a time and show before and after comparisons of data. Try to get as close as possible to 100 percent of the data from patients who fall into the category being studied. Use that data to chart the results and show change in that specific indicator over time. Graph the mean as a single line with upper and lower control limits to show statistically valid data. This statistical process control (SPC) chart shows whether the data is getting better or worse in a simple, easily understood fashion.

### Step Three: Create a Balance Sheet

If the project is to be a financial success, forecasting is required. The savings achieved must pay for the new process implementation, a portion of the improvement research cost, and provider incentives. A balance sheet or profit-and-loss statement that shows reimbursement, projected volume, and unit-specific cost can be used to forecast these costs. This step is the most commonly omitted in feasibility projections, even though it is critical if the partnership hopes to prove economic benefits of improvement.

To start, construct a table that lists the costs in the left-hand column and the benefits in the right-hand column. Start with the projected dollars saved as basic to the project, but also consider any intangible benefits such as increased physician participation in change and improved trust. If these issues are important, they will need to be quantified as part of the return on investment (ROI). Intangibles can be measured with a survey of the physicians' attitude about change. For example, an analysis of physician participation in meetings could be used to document cooperation.

### Step Four: Create a List of Milestones

Outline the measurable milestones as a way to define progress. Project how long it will take to gather the baseline data. Clarify who in administration is responsible for communicating with the physicians, how the key indicators will be tracked and in whose computer, and when the results will be printed graphically to document the change.

The final milestone is always the financial accounting for success. Certain financial standards must be met or the project will either be abandoned or rolled out at a painfully slow pace. These standards are

- Aligned incentives

- Tracking of savings needed to cover the cost of the CPI

- The cost of the reimbursing physicians for their time spent on the study

- Allocation of savings for physician reward

Successful CPI efforts typically project up to 50 percent of the savings to be retained by the system as an investment to support future work, 25 percent to be used to complete the study, and the remaining 25 percent to be used for physician incentives.

Physicians find the predictability of financial success within meaningful CPI projects easier to calculate with experience. This dimension is critical because it allows for specific gain sharing regardless of the reimbursement method. The key success factor is the forecast. When gains are predicted and achieved they serve to motivate. Now the team can ask: "Is changing care the right thing to do?"

## Operationalizing CPI

A description of how to move from determining feasibility to actually operationalizing CPI is described next. This implementation plan evolved from MRM's efforts to duplicate the excellent results achieved at IHC in organizations with inadequate information support.

Most of the hospitals that MRM has helped to implement CPI did not have extensive electronic support. Additional steps were added to the first phase to aid in gathering reliable data. Guidance for those working in support roles has also proved beneficial.

This model works because it is scientifically rigorous. This model and other simpler models are based on quality control and analysis theory. When deciding on how complex a CPI effort will be, remember that simplification is done at the expense of some scientific integrity. A simpler approach can be very effective; the determining factor should be how reliable the evidence needs to be. If it is a simple variation study of an accepted procedure with no incentives, excess rigor is an unnecessary expense and may slow the process down (or even kill it). Overly complex CPI efforts are often the cause of failed efforts in disease state management.

If the CPI project is the subject of a physician incentive proposal—that is, where exact success is being equated to dollars
returned to the physicians—the scientific accuracy of the project
becomes more critical. The AIMS approach—assessment, implementation, measurement, and sustaining the gains—is the backbone of classic CPI efforts. The model should be managed by a
well-educated team that is capable of using physicians as consultants. CPI programs fail because there is no accountability to
achieve each of these steps on a timeline. In the past, quality improvement professionals were rare and failure was common. The
AIMS model will now take the growing number of improvement
teams through a process that will succeed (see Exhibit 5.1).

## Keys to AIMS Success

By checking off each step as it is done and by establishing an accelerated timeline, the AIMS approach can ensure success. The only way
to fail is to omit steps or to slow down enough to lose momentum.

### Phase One: Assessment

*Step one: Establish a team and select a clinical area to improve.* The
first step is to review the feasibility report. Select a specific clinical
area that has proven to be feasible and then review the possible
team members. Next, find out who is truly interested in being
involved. This process should be easy if the feasibility analysis just
described has been done properly. The team needs to learn about
the CPI model in order to be fully invested in the project. Once the
staff has been educated about CPI and some enthusiasm has been
elicited, a mission or opportunity statement is drafted. Give a title
to the project that anyone can understand at a glance. The team
should set some basic rules for conducting the team meeting.

*Step two: Create a flow chart of the process.* This process will help
determine the relative importance of specific steps. This often helps

**Exhibit 5.1. The MRM AIMS Model.**

Overview of the CPI Process

Phase 1. Assessment

- Establish a team and select a clinical area to improve
- Create a flow of the process
- Prioritize the opportunities to improve
- Identify inputs and outputs and expectations
- Determine what can be measured and start to build an analysis plan
- Create a data sheet to retrieve key quality data
- Identify key processes with quality tools
- Refine self-coding data sheet
- Improve your data implementation effort
- Finalize your plan to analyze data
- Analyze the data
- Select the processes to be improved

Phase 2. Implementation

- Create the improvement plan
- Plan clinical education and process tracking
- Implement the improvement plan

Phase 3. Measurement

- Analyze the new data and results of the process change
- Measure the return on investment

Phase 4. Sustaining the Gains

- Continue and expand CPI efforts—Institute
- Integrate CPI projects throughout the system

clarify the exact opportunity for improvement and defines the data elements that need collecting.

*Step three: Prioritize the opportunities to improve.* The team defines the highest priority opportunity for improvement and the key factors that will need to change via cause-and-effect logic. For example, the timing of antibiotics was found to be the key step necessary to reduce postoperative wound infections, so the team focused on that step.

*Step four: Identify inputs, outputs, and expectations.* Process, output, expectation, and measurement provide the links between key people involved in the delivery of care and the measurable outcomes that will confirm success or failure of the project. Begin tracking data collection at this point. This step is difficult for many teams because they either don't like data in general or they begin to see that measurable expectations to achieve the process improvement leads to accountability that has never before existed. Creating a quality committee to manage this step helps.

*Step five: Determine what can be measured and start to build an analysis plan.* At this point, the team must learn about data tools and the graphic display of data. Data analysis should be kept simple enough to use off-the-shelf statistical software to display graphs that prove the validity of the data. For example, statistical process control (SPC) charts are run charts with upper and lower control limits. These are helpful for seeing variation and trends. The SPC chart shown in Figure 5.1 shows a process that is much better than the national average and has no outlier points that exceed the upper and lower control limits. Although there is still variation, these data are within the control limits, thus indicating that the process is under control.

*Step six: Create a data sheet to retrieve key quality data.* Once the analysis plan is agreed on, the data should be entered into a database with data sheets specifying exactly what data will be used for the study. An example for the disease state management of asthma

**Figure 5.1. Sample Statistical Process Control Chart.**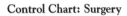

**Control Chart: Surgery**

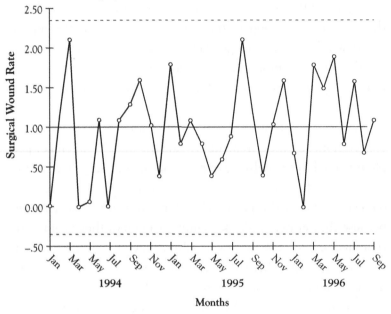

— Surgical Wound Rate
- - - UCL = 2.3528
— Average = .9958
- - - LCL = .3613

Reproduced courtesy of Nebraska Methodist Hospital.

can be found in Chapter Ten (Figure 10.2). Often this data can be used for other studies, so electronic support for some key components of data collection should be used. If the decision is made to automate data collection, these key components will eventually support an electronic medical record. At that level of information support, the software can be tied into a growing clinical informatics platform.

*Step seven: Identify key processes with quality tools.* Via statistical software, the quality team analyzes the data and creates graphic displays to look for variation. The data collection process and the original assumptions about the study are reevaluated. Wide variation that shows individuals that are more than two standard deviations off of the mean usually indicates bad data and may require adjustments in both collection and the analysis plan. A variable computation key can help describe a cause-and-effect relationship involving financial and clinical issues that could lead to incentives. For example, the mathematical formula defining the exact use of variables as they are employed to compute new variables, such as cost per unit of care, need to be written down and agreed upon. This is a critical step, especially when aligned incentives are based on these computations.

*Step eight: Refine self-coding data sheets.* After completing step seven, the team can review and refine the data sheet that describes all the needed data. If indicators are listed on the sheet that are not needed to solve the problem at hand, this is the time to remove them. Write up a data management book that documents the steps you have taken to improve the data so that others can solve problems quickly in the future.

*Step nine: Improve your data collection effort.* Implementation of more complex data collection can now go forward after an assessment of data entering, transfer, and analysis. Refine the data management instruction manual to describe a method for electronic entry of data with timelines, including milestones for collection, analysis, and display. Discussions are then held to set a plan to implement collection of data on time. An intervention plan should be discussed at this point if data collection is falling behind.

*Step ten: Finalize your plan to analyze data.* Revisit the plan for analysis after refining data-entering plans. Your plan should include

- A goal for data input

- A plan for computations, including factors that affect computed results

- An overview of the types of display of data to be used

- Clear study questions that are being answered by the analysis

Upon completing this step, outline a formal agreement on the framework for analyzing software development and reporting. A timeline for completing the project should now include the addition of any new software development time, new data collection, new analysis, and new development of reports with graphic display.

*Step eleven: Analyze the data.* Once the data are collected, the process of organizing the patient base and the number of patients begins. Unexpected key contributing variables may appear, as will apparent interrelationships between variables. Another possibility is that the data will demonstrate such wide variation that the stability of the clinical process must be questioned. What emerges from the data has the potential to upset physicians, so it is important to establish new processes linked with a support structure that can implement change and reward new success quickly. As physicians see large differences in reward, those who are not eligible for the bonus due to poor compliance with a protocol begin to pay attention. This first completed analysis creates a baseline from which to improve. Peer support can then be used to affect physician behavior.

*Step twelve: Select the processes to be improved.* The physicians involved in the study need to agree on a plan for change based on the data. A physician champion invites peer feedback and discussion. Possible strategies to carry out new protocol steps can be briefly outlined at this juncture. The team must focus on facts that reflect how change will benefit the participants in the improvement project. For example, if a projection of successful implementation can be made showing the physicians a potential bonus amount that will be provided when they reach 75 percent of the benchmark results, successful process improvement is likely.

## Phase Two: Implementation

*Step one: Create the improvement plan.* The first step to timely CPI implementation is often the installation of an action plan for a simple protocol. Techniques to achieve cooperative agreement among peers vary, but this step usually leads the list of CPI challenges. Keep a record of how the team of physician champions achieves agreement at this stage to guide others with subsequent efforts. Eventually, a peer discussion manual will emerge. Once a plan is accepted by those who must use it, the previous steps have achieved a fair amount of physician and nurse feedback without wasting the provider's time. The implementation plan should clarify what exact agreements the providers have made for change, the role of support personnel needed to facilitate change and collect data, and the agreed-upon analysis, graphic display, and reporting methods.

*Step two: Plan clinical education and process tracking.* After the action plan is set, education and process tracking begin. The education process reinforces the need for successful implementation. It should be repetitive and managed on a timeline. Many organizations create an institute to formalize this step. The larger the CPI undertaking, the more complex and formal this process must become.

*Step three: Implement the improvement plan.* This is the stage at which an organization's support structure is tested. Formal change management includes education on the process of change itself. Accountability becomes critical here. Many organizations discover that the support is inadequate and needs to be reinforced. Ask personnel to write down the barriers encountered, so that the team can redesign the support effort. Failing to implement CPI plans properly is the problem with most failed CPI efforts. The next chapter on high performance will offer more detailed solutions regarding implementation.

### Phase Three: Measurement

*Step one: Analyze the new data and results of the process change.* After change is in place, the team needs to assess the assumptions used to justify the study. Success or failure should be judged by the validity of the original assumptions and the implementation effort. Track the percentage of process change achieved as well as the percentage of steps accomplished within the timelines. When problems are encountered, a new protocol or support mechanism may need to be structured and implemented. Whenever possible, create single-entry electronic support that remains in place for ongoing improvement efforts that will follow the study.

*Step two: Measure the return on investment (ROI).* Once the clinical change is clear, the team can calculate the cost of the project as well as the return on investment. This step requires a correlation between the needed financial data and specific units of care that changed because of the study. Look especially for unintended consequences like cost shifting, as decreased costs in one part of the continuum of care often increase costs somewhere else in the system. For example, shortening the length of a hospital stay always increases the need for home care and support from the doctor's office. Measuring the cause-and-effect relationships of change in terms of cost and revenue becomes critical.

The financial calculations need to be adjusted for the various methods of reimbursement. Each organization involved in the same study may be paid under fee-for-service, per diem, capitation, or global payment. When these methods are all present in the same system, they are always in conflict. In other words, the change will not have the same financial result for each method. Some reimbursements may actually have a negative financial impact when other methods are providing reward. If a risk pool or direct risk contract is in place, the plan to distribute savings after balancing the profit and loss data will depend on these calculations. The formulas for these calculations should have been agreed to in writing during the feasibility analysis.

Assuming some contracts reflect fee-for-service and some are capitated, calculate the savings created for the third party contrasted to physicians' incentive bonuses as a powerful exercise. Shown graphically, physicians can emphasize whether improvements in care are rewarding the providers or creating an economic opportunity for a third party that removes economic resources from the health care partnership. The team should determine whether this type of information will be inflammatory or motivational, but the quality improvement steering committee should at least see the reports.

### Phase Four: Sustaining the Gains

*Step one: Institutionalize.* The most practical method to improve the CPI ability of the new partnerships is to institutionalize it. Chapter Nine describes an improvement office to spread the CPI philosophy and support projects for years to come. Once the necessary support is in place, the data collection analysis and reporting will be uniform and standard. The office or institute will be a revenue center with adequate resources and authority to carry out the research that has been described in this chapter.

*Step two: Integrate CPI projects throughout the system.* To achieve full integration, the preceding steps are organized electronically. From there, the structure and focus of a relational clinical data repository will emerge systemwide. With the capability for electronic medical records, CPI efforts can be expanded. Knowledge alerts or smart computers can be used to remind physicians to use key process steps 100 percent of the time. The acceptance of these electronic helpers is greatly enhanced if they support economic reward. Coupled with aligned incentive strategies, these kinds of projects can be a powerful force to integrate the new partnerships.

## Critical Elements

- Getting executive leadership to believe that CPI proves that a desired outcome can be achieved by consistently implementing a best-clinical-process step.

- Teaching CQI/TQM methods applied to direct clinical care.

- Agreeing on clinical and financial indicator measurements.

- Using the literature to determine what should be improved and which step should be measured to get the greatest success.

- Doing a feasibility analysis before getting started. This requires

    A clear opportunity statement for improvement

    Unit-based cost analysis

    Financial projections for improvement

    Data management and analysis

    Simple, focused CPI

    Demonstrated relationship with previous work

    Physician champions

    CPI teams

    Accountable implementation on a timeline

    Proven benefits of process change

- Conducting the CPI project.

    Do the assessment

    Implement CPI

    Measure results

    Sustain the gains

- Rewarding success once the improvements demonstrate savings remains critical.

## CPI Becomes a Way of Thinking One Physician at a Time

Kenny knew there was something wrong. He had been waiting for the medication to arrive for more than thirty minutes when the anesthesiologist said, "Look, I'm going to have to bump your case, with or without the antibiotics."

"What is that supposed to mean?"

Dr. Green glared at Kenny. "You aren't the only physician, and this delay isn't acceptable. All of the surgeons don't even use prophylactic antibiotics with laparoscopy. This case won't take as long as you've been messing around waiting for pharmacy."

Kenny said, "Just relax, George."

"I can't relax. You decide, we go now, or I call for the next case and you go to the end of the day."

Kenny knew that Dr. Green was serious.

The circulating nurse, Karen, also heard the discussion. She was uncomfortable because she was the one responsible for logging the time the drug was given.

"This is very unusual Dr. Green. The pharmacy usually stocks the OR for the cases the night before. The admitting nurse should have recognized the problem as soon as she came on duty."

Kenny interrupted, "Well, I can't just skip the medication and I can't cancel the case."

"Well, you can't bump every case that follows yours by waiting for an hour after I give the antibiotic."

Kenny stepped toward Dr. Green, "Wait, the next case is also mine and it's a simple D&C. No antibiotic indicated and the patient is already here."

Kenny turned to Karen, the circulating nurse, "If you help get the patient moving, I'll get the pharmacy going and I can give the antibiotic." He turned to Dr. Green, "George, if you'll start the IV, I'll get the medication and Karen can get the next patient. By the time this patient is in the room, the antibiotic will be on board. We can do the second case first and the incision time should be exactly one hour post-antibiotics."

Kenny pointed to the pharmacy stocks, "Karen, be sure to get the rest of your meds lined up."

"Already done. My earlier call should have the ball rolling by now."

Dr. Green just stared. He always got angry when the first case was facing a delay. "OK."

Kenny shook Green's hand, "Thanks George, I owe you!"

"You certainly do."

Kenny smiled at Karen as she replied, "I'll find out what's going on."

"Thanks Karen. I'm glad you've got this prophylactic antibiotic project in place. I can't remember my last post-op infection on a routine case, and it's really the patient that benefits."

They turned to walk down the hall to preop.

"I remember one case where the patient ended up with peritonitis and an abscess, all of which started with a routine tubal sterilization. Best care demands these antibiotics. Thanks for helping with Dr. Green."

"I'll change the room, call for a D&C pack, and cover the laparoscopy equipment. We'll be back on schedule in no time."

This chapter has briefly addressed the strategy and requirements to use CPI as a method to achieve positive change. These steps are a critical means of organizing and using data systems. However, compulsive implementation of a proven structure is necessary to achieve accountability and reward wherever aligned incentives exist. In Chapter Six the human performance issues will be addressed, as well as the ability of a group of professionals to work together effectively as a team to add even more opportunity for success.

# 6

# The Fourth Dimension
## High-Performance Teams Through Interdependence and Learning

In the last chapter, the third dimension, clinical process improvement, was explored from a structural and operational perspective. This chapter looks at the fourth dimension, high performance and cooperation, and how it can be integrated with the first three dimensions, integrated information exchange, aligned incentives, and clinical process improvement. High performance and cooperation are needed to build the culture that can support the first three dimensions. With cooperation within the clinical group providing care, the family, and the community, an entirely new approach to health care partnerships emerges. Though the technical potential to improve care and reward physicians may be in place, the new practice must overcome physician infighting and controlling behavior. This chapter focuses on the need for new physician leadership and offers an approach to overcoming barriers to cooperation.

To transform a practice professionals need a higher level of interaction and team performance than has been necessary in the past. Physicians who work interdependently create more clinical improvements and more rewards. The major challenge for the new practice partnership is abandoning old control and authority-driven practice habits.

## Training in Cooperation
## Is the Foundation for Change

Physicians, possibly more than any other type of provider, must be
formally educated before they will change their behavior. Chris
Argyris has written a great deal about defensive routines that are
common to high-performing, intelligent people (Argyris, 1995).
These intelligent individuals make complex, rapid, correct decisions
constantly. They need to consider the cause-and-effect relationship of decisions but there is no time to question the validity of
each of the assumptions made for each decision. To question even
one step in the decision-making process would be to falter, and high-
performing physicians don't have time to falter or hesitate. Physicians subconsciously believe they are always right—the only way a
flow state of peak performance becomes possible (Csikszentmihalyi,
1990). These high-performance learning parameters must be kept in
mind as physicians are educated to change a practice pattern that
has become a habit.

Physicians, like all independent high performers, are uncomfortable abandoning behavior that has served them well in the past.
For example, even when innovation is proven to get better results
than old performance patterns, it is common for the innovation to
be resisted or ignored. Simply giving this new information to the
physicians may not convince them to question their habitualized
personal decisions because it is so comforting to stay with what they
believe to be true.

Behavioral psychology explains why many protocols and national benchmarks that document the ability to improve outcomes
will have little impact on physician behavior. By far, the majority
of physicians have missed the potential described in the last two
chapters because they just keep doing what past experience has
taught them is "practicing good medicine." Without data and facts,
physicians were forced to assume their approach was the best way
to do things. To lose this confidence would have compromised per-

formance. New partnerships should keep this in mind as they establish strategies that are dependent on new cooperative, coordinated delivery models. Even with the reward, creating an acceptance for change remains the greatest challenge to implementing case management and clinical redesign. Physicians' tendency to rebel against change has been ignored in the approach most have taken to improving clinical performance. Resistance to change needs to be managed if change is to occur.

## A Theory Physicians Can Trust

Self-directed learning is the primary means for adults to facilitate change (Knowles, 1998). An objective, constructive, and timely feedback process can bring about behavioral change. The most important success factor is a theory of improving clinical behavior and performance that gives physicians the opportunity to prove or disprove what works.

The theoretical basis for training in cooperative physician leadership must include both technical performance issues (productivity, accuracy, and speed of implementation) and human performance issues (reaching agreement, smoothing out the delivery or transfer of care, and learning from experience). Training to achieve cooperation must also use a common language that can bridge the wide ethnic and socioeconomic boundaries that define the physician patient encounter (Prather, Blake, and Mouton, 1990a).

Medical Resource Management's experience in training physicians has proven that they resist psychological and "touchy-feely" language. In addition, for this effort to directly influence patient care it needs to address the broad differences in knowledge that exist between those providing and those receiving care.

### Lessons from Malpractice Litigation

A physician-owned insurance company utilized a behavioral science model to train practicing physicians as the basis for an experiment to reduce the dollars lost and the frequency of malpractice claims for physicians. A performance improvement model from outside the field of medicine was selected. This model was based on cooperative decision-making and conflict-solving training models grounded in organizational psychology. The training was then delivered via proven, experience-based, adult education techniques (Kolb, 1984).

This new experimental model focused on patient care and offered the physicians an opportunity to evaluate cooperation as a technique to achieve informed consent and patient compliance. A series of competitive team exercises provided the basis for training. As performance improved on a given team, physicians taught each other the skills they used to succeed, thus reinforcing the concept of cooperation. The team that came in last was motivated to use the new skills to gain a competitive advantage over the other teams. In a short time, the physicians actually taught each other to shift their values from control and authority toward learning. This model proves the value of cooperation over control, paternalism, compromise, and avoidance. When surveyed, physicians in practice preferred the value of cooperation (Prather, Blake, and Mouton, 1990b). One challenge facing these physicians was retaining the skills once they returned to work. Actually using cooperative techniques to resolve differences of opinion, especially under stress, is hard work.

This high-performance model is an application of Dr. Jane Mouton and Robert Blake's work in organizational development, called Grid™ theory (Blake and Mouton, 1968). Grid™ theory has been validated in a wide cross section of cultures around the world, thus making it the perfect candidate for a model to use with the wide ethnic and educational background of physicians and patients. The Grid™ model, when adapted to medicine by Medical Resource Management (MRM), had the positive impact on physicians' behavior that the liability carriers had hoped for.

### Learning from the Airline Industry

This unique physician training model, which has continued to evolve, most recently under VHA's endorsement, is now called

Achieving High-Performance Relationships (AHPR). The Grid™ theory applies the training of jet airliner pilots to the high-risk world of physician practice.

In 1979, NASA research showed that the majority of fatal air crashes were caused by human error. To address the economic and human losses of in-flight catastrophes, United Airlines partnered with Mouton and Blake's company, Scientific Methods, Inc. (SMI), to test their theory. This joint effort began a training tradition that would go on to revolutionize the education of airline pilots. The effort spawned the term *cockpit resource management*, or CRM, now widely used in the industry (Blake and Mouton, 1984).

All airlines used flight simulators and a rigorous military type of training to improve pilots' technical skills. Until performance theory and adult education techniques were merged into the repetitive, videotaped training sessions of CRM, little improvement over national norms was seen in pilot performance via the traditional approach (Lavber, 1980). Prior to application of CRM to United Airlines, the pilots' performance statistics were similar among all major carriers. After several years of this training in cooperative decision making and high performance, United reduced measured error rates in routine flight three-fold compared with the rest of the industry (*The Cockpit*, 1986). United pilots went on to fly seven million air hours without a fatal accident. The rest of the industry averaged 1.5 million air hours flown for every hull loss (serious accident) logged. The FAA was so impressed with these statistics they made CRM-type training a requirement for licensing pilots (National Transportation Safety Board, 1985, pp. 1–5).

The first application of this high-performance model of training for physicians was never published, because the study results were not intended for public review. But the first three years of data did demonstrate a statistically significant decline in dollars lost and claims frequency for those physicians trained, compared to all other physicians insured. Ten years later the data still demonstrates a significant difference in these parameters. Although the research did not include measures of reduced error, the improvements were achieved among a group of physicians with multiple previous lawsuits. The long-term impact on this group of physicians was very significant to the liability carrier.

## The MRM Method

The Medical Resource Management method of training evolved from the CRM experience. Just like CRM, MRM includes a very formal study of cooperation. Physicians study the theory of behavioral style in *Behavioral Types: The Art of Patient Management* (Prather, Blake, and Mouton, 1990a). Where pilot training uses the records of an airliner crash to model simulations, the physician training can draw on the circumstances that are felt to be at the root of medical catastrophes and malpractice litigation. This approach is now being tailored to more common medical situations that the literature indicates can be improved. This method of teaching high performance has been introduced into several medical school curriculums. For example, the University of Eastern Carolina Medical Center has a long-term plan to create an integrated health care system. The new partnership model they are creating is centered at Pitt County Memorial Hospital (PCMH) in Greenville, North Carolina. Their plan is to make high performance and cooperation a formal part of the medical curriculum from the first day of orientation to graduation.

To ensure a cultural change across an entire health care partnership group, this health care system realized that they would need to train administrators to partner with physicians. Nurses were also trained, thereby completing the high-performance training loop.

### Improving Performance in ICUs

Physician performance training by using videotapes can improve performance in the intensive care unit (ICU) (Goldman, 1985, p. 173). Recurrent training in these programs has increased actual survival rates in cardiopulmonary resuscitation (CPR). Video training can also improve day-to-day ICU outcomes but is rarely used in this manner.

MRM training is based on the CRM philosophy and utilizes interactive video simulations and videotaped interviews. Educational sessions focus on known cooperative high-performance solutions to real problems. The ability to reduce errors with this type of education is demonstrated through a comparison of error rates before and after training via the CPI methods described in Chapter Five. Success depends on high performance. The physician's ability to resolve conflict quickly through interpersonal communication decreases error. Performance improvement is achieved through cooperative and efficient conflict resolution followed by learning. These performance skills are rapidly becoming targets for aggressively cooperative partnerships that realize the importance of improved medical performance. Partnerships committed to providing the best care are becoming more focused on reducing errors made during actual process steps of care. This trend will increase, since errors in patient care are now being more widely documented and reported (Carothers, 1998, p. 104).

### The Pressure of Public Comparisons

Comparisons of hospitals and medical group practices are being made by the National Committee for Quality Accreditation and the Joint Commission on Accreditation of Healthcare Organizations. Soon, the American Medical Association's National Patient Safety Foundation will publish their own comparisons. This group's website address says it all, www.mederrors.org.

These organizations are already making preliminary comparisons of the error rates of clinicians and hospitals. These comparisons will become increasingly detailed as tracking and dissemination become easier and more efficient. As public comparisons become more accessible, physician stress will go up. Physician cooperation will be difficult at first, but the fear of being in the lower half of the data will motivate physicians to change. Groups who use cooperation to guide this change will find that it is a powerful tool within new partnerships striving to improve outcomes.

The success of formal efforts to reduce errors by using CPI has shown that average care across the country in certain diagnostic related groups (DRGs) is failing to meet the new standards of best care (Gerety, 1994, p. 29). CPI alone is not enough. A new type of training is also needed. The skills of active listening, focused attention, and delegating tasks can be taught and evaluated as physicians attempt to use new skills in confidential video simulations.

The majority of caregivers in America have not begun formal improvement training to reduce the errors of human memory. The question facing integrated systems is, "How do we motivate physicians to lead this change?" These partnerships are also asking, "Is being average a failure if it can be proven that some systems are capable of reducing human error and improving outcomes two or three-fold over our results?" This situation is not unlike the Federal Aviation Agency's (FAA's) when the error rates in groups of pilots improved and the FAA decided to require a new type of performance training, thus moving an entire industry to a higher level of expectation and outcome in the process.

The new expectations of the public will inspire physicians who are committed to the new practice of medicine. Other physicians will feel threatened by the public's expectations. As the new practices come together in partnerships that can participate in information-driven cooperative models of care, groups of physicians will teach each other to improve even as they hold each other accountable to change. These practices realize that it is far better to create this type of success than to be unfavorably compared to it.

If medicine followed the policy of the FAA, MRM-type training would become a requirement of medical licensure much in the same way CRM-type training became a requirement for maintaining a jet airline pilot's license. The evolution of this requirement will not affect physicians in the new partnerships because they will already be trained and providing the type of care that sets benchmarks. As researchers describe their clinical successes through higher performance, these new partnerships will already be redesigning and implementing new clinical processes to ensure that they keep ahead of the curve.

## Integrating High Performance into the Practice

Under the most successful practice philosophies, cooperative group performance will replace independent, fragmented models of care. The old model did not require physicians to communicate, cooperate, or formally train to prevent errors. In the present information era, physicians must facilitate information transfer between providers. Ignoring this complex process allows errors to go undetected and therefore unprevented. Joint decision making and team-based delivery of care are faster and less error prone than fragmented, independent models. For example, a focus on communication can eliminate lost lab work, call schedules, and phone messages. Physicians can evaluate the process of communication in a variety of stressful circumstances in short weekly sessions. A small group of committed individuals can begin to help each other without malice but with openness and candor.

The training is done in small, accountable groups, which make trust easier to achieve and maintain. Physician leaders working within these new partnerships are able to resolve conflict. They also learn from day-to-day experience. Implementing the technical aspects of CPI is more about high levels of cooperation than improvement theory. The new partnership becomes a practice accountable for quality (PAQ). The office manager is responsible for surveying progress at the end of the day to evaluate physicians' effectiveness, level of cooperation, and satisfaction with the clinical team's performance. Physicians survey themselves at the end of the month to evaluate the financial impact of their improvement strategy. Physician leaders will achieve higher personal satisfaction in the practice of medicine once they cooperate more formally.

The new practice of medicine approaches health care in a way that is professionally superior to the old, "more is better" model. Success is the result of making a contribution under a clear strategy. It requires focused training and uses facts to prove that clinical success has been achieved. Success is linked to widespread communication, so the practice can learn from itself. Once this new capacity for change has been reached by a group of trusted colleagues, the opportunity described in the previous chapter becomes a reality.

## Critical Elements

- A theory base for behavioral change that physicians will accept.

- A recurrent training model to reinforce high performance.

- Physician motivation to take training in group cooperation.

- Videotaped simulations of conflict resolution tracking process steps linked to performance.

- Comparisons of clinical outcomes measures before and after training.

- Bonus incentives based on the savings that result from cooperation.

- Survey of provider satisfaction and perception of cooperation.

- Open dialogues on the uncomfortable issues that prevent trust.

- Deciding what needs to change, and then helping the physicians guide process redesign with data.

- Surveys of the practice's level of cooperation.

- Tracking accountability for the new roles needed to cross the old silos.

### NewMed Physician Leaders Teach Cooperation by Example

Kenny looked up from his case and saw the persistent, angry expression of Dr. Green. "Come on, let's all just lighten up a bit."

Karen, the circulating nurse, jotted something on a piece of paper as she walked around the table behind Dr. Green. She held it up so Kenny could read the message. "Open-ended questions!

Kenny appreciated the reminder. "How is it going up there, George?"

"Don't worry about what's going on up here, just keep working so we can make up the time. Jamison follows you, and you know who he is going to blame for any delay."

Kenny recalled seeing this kind of conflict on one of the video training tapes. He actually wanted to improve his relationship with George, but how? Delays were almost always preventable and now that anesthesia was on an incentive bonus for turn-around time, Dr. Green's anxiety was partly dollars and cents.

"George, about this morning. What do you think the OR team could have done to prevent the delay?"

"Don't ask me, the team is supposed to get the drugs to me on time. I'm not the problem here."

Kenny felt the old tension and considered giving up.

Karen quickly interjected, "The problem this morning was in pharmacy. We are tracking which process steps got dropped, and this one was definitely pharmacy."

"I didn't say who's to blame," Kenny replied. "But, what I'm trying to find out is how I can be more effective if this sort of problem occurs in the future. George, what would you have done in my shoes?"

"Nothing, nothing."

"No, really. You and I could follow up on this. We could get our departments to agree on some set policies about moving the order of patients when the antibiotics aren't available. I don't want to search for a new solution to this kind of conflict with every anesthesiologist on staff, and you don't want a different response from every surgeon."

"That's true," agreed George.

"Where would you start?"

Silence filled the room. It seemed like an hour before George replied, "Well, our department could write that kind of policy. I think the anesthesiologists should have the privilege of bumping cases when the patients are not prepped and we have a busy day."

"That's not exactly what I asked, George! It's not about you or I having power over the other, it's about a better flow of patient care."

"Excuse me. You two aren't alone here. All solutions don't require a physician's order."

"That's right. Karen and the rest of the staff could have the authority to solve these problems before they put us in conflict."

"What's wrong with conflict? You will never get everyone to agree. Kenny, you're always overthinking everything."

"Well, the real problem with conflict, Dr. Green, is delay. If you and your colleagues go through the process we all went through today very often, it probably costs you money."

Dr. Green established eye contact for the first time, as he looked up from the monitors. "That's a good point."

"George, how do we get this ball rolling?"

Kenny knew he had found the bridge. He knew that George needed to be in the driver's seat. Kenny could give up control because he knew the quality improvement team could implement a structured flow of patients in the OR if anesthesia got behind it.

"Well, I can present it to my department but the surgeons are the real problem."

"Don't be so sure, George. This effort may not fall victim to more of the old OR battles. We all have a lot to gain from improving patient flow. Time is money to us all."

Kenny turned to Karen. "Your OR team will be behind you and we can prove whether your decisions get implemented within the first month of the improvement project."

"Great!"

Kenny nodded to George and said thank you to Karen. Kenny was helping everyone around him move in a positive direction but he wasn't using control. He was listening and being genuinely cooperative and committed to positive change. His impact was felt in the OR across a time-honored and traditional battle zone.

This chapter has reviewed the principles of teaching high performance with suggestions for interactive physician training within the practice setting. As new levels of cooperation and high performance are reached, the first three dimensions, information management, economic reward, and quality improvement, become tools that distinguish the new partnerships. Chapter Seven explains how to use these skills to engage the patient and family as true partners in the new cooperation described here. Reinforcing the family's role in health management is described as the fifth dimension of the new physician leadership.

# The Fifth Dimension
## Partnering with the Family

The previous chapter emphasized the importance of overcoming resistance to change to allow for the interdependence and cooperation needed for improvement strategies. In this chapter, the commitment to cooperative accountability is extended to the patient and the patient's family as a means of implementing disease state management and decreasing the need for treatment.

## Family Support Systems

It has long been assumed that the social support of the patient's family (or support group) is beneficial to treatment. Now this impact can be measured through a more expansive and inclusive approach to disease state management (Davis and Hamill, 1997, p. 48). Diabetes care provides a good example. Without adequate family or social support, a child with diabetes is admitted regularly to the hospital and often faces life-threatening situations. Prevention of prolonged and frequent hospitalization for all patients with diabetes not only creates significant direct savings, but also prevents long-term complications such as renal failure and blindness (Diabetes Control and Complications Trial Research Group, 1996, p. 1409). Education and home health visits are used to create family support, thus improving the quality of life for these chronically ill patients dramatically (Butler and others, 1998, p. 63). By committing to cooperation through use of CPI measures under aligned incentives and good information management, the new practice partnership can quantify the amount of money it takes to educate the family of an individual with this condition. With unit-based cost accounting, the costs of care can be shown to be reduced beyond the cost of patient and family education (Dougherty and others, 1999, p. 122). The new partnership uses the savings to reward the practice and reinvest in the community.

### Identifying Support Systems

In terms of support, the "family" is not limited to direct or even biological relations. Volunteers, church groups, and social support agencies can serve as family. The *family* can be defined as a group of people who care for each other and who share a bond based on some type of mutual dependence. The key factor is that family members interact with each other on a daily basis and have a commitment to be together during the foreseeable future, even if it includes illness. The only requirement for the new practice is that family members provide a structure within which effective disease state management, self-diagnosis, and self-care can happen.

Masters-trained nurse clinicians are an important link in the family care model. Nurse clinicians take medical care out of the office and into the home. They work directly with the family and outline family protocols, thus extending the practice's reach. As the new practices formalize and implement family-focused delivery of care, dieticians, occupational therapists, social workers, and other educators will become important members of the cooperative care management team. Partnerships in family-focused care demonstrate that patients and providers have the ability and the need to partner together in care.

The goal of family-focused care is to keep the patient and the family at the center of the care systems that support them. For example, in a mature, well-educated family that is supported by a well-functioning system, even patients with chronic illness are able to care for themselves. Family members remind patients how to walk through numerous self-care tasks, and they also maintain a home treatment log for documentation. If patients cannot care for themselves with family support, nurses, educators, and primary care physicians need to become involved. These providers offer the first line of care through triage that directs simple treatment with education. The patient is directed to the specialist physician only when the highest level of knowledge regarding an organ-specific disease is required.

### Tracking the Family's Success

In the intact family, where the majority of patients spend most of their lives, patients are educated to create a healthy mind and body. This can include a wellness or fitness approach with specific modification for chronic illness. Even with good education and support, however, not everyone will succeed at learning self-care. The new practice will need to monitor the family's ability to participate in these self-care plans. For example, a family member must maintain the home treatment log. If a family cannot remember to record daily treatments, they are probably not implementing the proper care. The home treatment log is a useful indicator as to how much support the patient is receiving.

### Adapting to the Family Style

Providers need to use the right type of education to affect widely diverse family environments. This requires both knowledge of human behavior and a formal plan to help a family function in a supportive manner. A dysfunctional family can tax the educational resources of even the most experienced nurses and educators. Fortunately, the majority of families are supportive and willing to learn.

To determine the right type of education, first perform a cultural evaluation of the primary support person in the patient's life. This can be accomplished with the same behavioral theory that providers use to design their own interdependent, high-performing teams. A medical team using high-performance training can use simulations of difficult situations to understand different family styles.

In an average family situation, the triage nurse creates a protocol in collaboration with the physicians who are responsible for care. The complexity of the self-care protocol is classified as either high or low, based on the number and complexity of decisions. Next, a check-off sheet is added to the patient's record that categorizes patients and family members with special needs. By separating the families into the broad categories of *compromising support, controlling support, avoiding support,* and *cooperating support,* the practice can go to work. Because each category of support requires a different approach, the triage nurse alerts the provider to special needs prior to the clinical visit. The following adjectives are typical of the different types of support. As a clear style of family support becomes obvious, different strategies can be put in place.

*Avoidance* families are resigned, have a wait-and-see attitude, are unresponsive, followers, tentative, passive, uninvolved, and unmotivated.

*Control* families often include perfectionists, have a know-it-all attitude, are quick to blame, patronizing, arrogant, overpowering, condescending, demanding, and impatient.

*Compromise* families are usually accommodating, negotiating, appreciative, agreeable, conforming, cautious, noncontroversial, supportive, and rationalizing.

*Cooperative* families are innovative, positive, confident, motivated, collaborative, open-minded, spontaneous, candid, responsive, and decisive.

The majority of patients fall into the *compromise* or average support category. The average family needs to be given clear instructions with education that starts with the first phone call. The goal of education is to move these traditional families from a compromise approach, where they will do some of what they are asked to do, to cooperation, at which point they really get involved. Once the practice has determined that the family is ready to take on an active role in self-care and self-screening, members of the family can even start to help others who lack family support. A plan is written down and this new supportive partner becomes part of the care plan. Follow-up ensures that cooperation has emerged. Families who are in the categories of avoiding or controlling support are approached with a different but specific plan based on what will work to meet their unique needs. This type of plan is usually the result of experience more than anything else. The challenge is learning the potential for support that exists within each family.

A family may give the provider clues when they bring a patient in. For example, a family member may say, "Well, we've been trying to get him to come in for months but he just wouldn't have it until he couldn't get out of bed yesterday." The triage nurse could then ask questions such as, "Who helps the patient at home? Who checks his medications? Who in the family could walk with him three times per week? What is in his refrigerator? What does he eat, and how often? How often does someone in the family visit him?" to learn more. The answers to these questions and the adjectives that describe the family's attitude become key to the patient's health and also reveal the style of family support.

The medical Grid™ theory of behavioral change is used by Medical Resource Management and more recently by VHA in the educational seminar "Achieving High Performance Relationships (AHPR)." It has proven to be a good tool to organize not only the organization's and physician's cooperation, but the needed family education as well. Because grid theory has been validated in virtually all ethnic groups, it is a good model to use here. Whatever theory is used to direct education, it must provide a clear screening method to recognize difficult family cultures throughout the system.

For example, the two most common difficult family cultures are those who want more control than is good for the patient and those who are in avoidance and won't even talk about the patient's needs. In both situations, specific agreed-upon strategies should tailor the approach. Behavioral theory can help the practice predict the compliance of the family to various approaches.

If a dominant family member is angry and controlling, then building a strong relationship with that person is a key strategy. A provider could ask, "What information do you need to have to feel comfortable with your role? You and I will need to manage this situation together." This question addresses their obvious need for control without directly confronting or challenging them. The provider needs to define the control that the family member requires so that the provider team can cooperate with the family. Based on what the family member says, the educator outlines specific steps to give this individual a clear role as a home care manager. The patient may also benefit from social counseling or classes in conflict resolution. It is often helpful to focus part of the patient education on how the patient can get the most support from these dominant family members. Though difficult to live with, controlling family members are often very good at ensuring compliance if given the right direction.

In the case of a family that is in denial or avoidance, the provider addresses the fears that make home care so threatening. Home health professionals demonstrate simple but helpful rituals to key family members.

The clinical team needs to recognize both the controlling and avoiding family support types, because their progress must be checked more often than other family types. If they have trouble complying with a written plan, more education than average is needed. Once a dysfunctional family is identified, volunteers from the community can be incorporated into the patient's support system, as long as they are formally trained in crisis management. In some cases, the family might disintegrate as a result of illness. In these situations, social work or psychological support is needed (Arpin and others, 1990, p. 373).

Fear of pain, suffering, and even death or just low self-esteem can make it difficult for families to learn new, more productive behaviors. Sometimes, a patient's family environment is uncaring or even dangerous. In these situations, social workers and even the police may need to be called upon. Whatever the strategy, the patient must invite and welcome the support provided and give their consent for the greater family support system to be part of their care plan. Although a formal written consent is not usually necessary, the provider team should attempt to document the patient's consent to anyone having information about their illness.

**Coping with the End of Life**

One of the most important times to involve a patient's family or friends in the care plan is at the end of life. When multiple chronic illnesses worsen, multiple acute episodes of illness treatment become necessary. At some point, the prognosis for even partial recovery will be unlikely. The new practice partnerships should take a formal approach about the ethics of medical decisions in these circumstances. Different strategies will be needed to help patients in all types of family support situations. A sound plan that balances human need with medical and technical ability must be devised to guide critical decisions about life support. As chronic illness becomes terminal, a care map that outlines what steps should be taken by whom offers relief to many families and patients. Some patients will require hospitalization to ease the dying process, but many people prefer the opportunity to die at home if they are assured of pain relief and social support (McCusker, 1985, p. 42). The growing use of hospice proves this (Paradis and others, 1983, p. 180). The family's comfort and level of understanding with the different options available often determines what care is provided.

The new partnerships strive to include the family much earlier than the usual hospice intervention. Because family-focused support often decreases the use of expensive, futile care, the practice should measure and document family satisfaction and the availability of care choices even if the patient has refused them.

The topic of ethics in medicine is a complex one and beyond the scope of this book. However, physicians of the new practice study ethics and human behavior to influence the whole patient, not just treating the patient's illness (La Puma, 1998).

### Training the Family

Group workshops are the most effective means of educating the family. Group workshops follow the model used in childbirth classes (Eliupoulus, 1997, p. 185). The family's primary caregiver attends with the patient, and an educator teaches everyone in the class about the disease. The support persons resolve their fears and concerns by sharing their personal concerns with others who are not medically trained. Warning signs, self-testing, techniques for doing lab tests, and methods of basic treatment are reviewed and practiced with the other participants and the educator.

For instance, parents learning to manage pediatric asthma and adult children learning to manage their parent's diabetes can both be taught in group classes. Schools, churches, and businesses can provide classrooms where the new practice educators provide the curriculum. Follow-up visits are used to answer questions and to explore the level of responsibility that the patient's support group wants to take on. It is surprising how much help some caring family members are able to provide in the home (Persily, 1996, p. 327). For example, terminal care, although stressful, is also seen as very important by families. Organizing care protocols and surrogate decision makers for the purpose of carrying out medical directives contained in living wills brings focus to everyone's role. Partnered with the physician, the family can give narcotics, change dressings, provide intervenous therapy, and generally relieve the suffering of the family member.

For home care models to be effective, the care plan must be followed and providers must be able to recognize unsafe care. For example, a domineering family member who takes on too much authority may decide that they know more than the doctors. But if a care map is used, filled out, and reviewed regularly, the care map will show whether a controlling family member is deviating from the plan. Families who fail to fill out the care map are either in the denial, avoidance, or control models of support. Patients in this situation should be shifted into more traditional care until social work and education can move the family to cooperation.

Holding regular family dialogues about the role of helping is one of the best methods for teaching the family to assume a role in patient care. Even this step requires a culturally specific approach so that the team can achieve the needed communication.

Technical support tools are appearing on the market that can help home educators and volunteers with the task of educating patients and families. An example is an interactive CD-ROM entitled *House Calls* that is manufactured by Adam's Graphics. This and other, similar tools prompt the user to ask the right questions when symptoms of illness or discomfort are present. These interactive programs can help volunteers teach mothers to find answers to simple but distressing health questions about their children. Instead of visiting the office, the mother either uses a CD-ROM herself or calls a trained educator with access to the technology.

Within self-diagnosis strategies, the new medicine uses personal health experts to assist individuals with triage protocols. For instance, personal health experts can take their laptop computers into the home to help elderly patients confused by the changes that occur with aging. These volunteers can download the information they gather to the practice via the Internet. In its most sophisticated application, an alerting system can call the physician when combinations of symptoms seem to warrant medical care. The practice needs systematically to record all the information gathered into a database. The technology and products to accomplish this level of care are already widely available. Many large HMOs have established self-care Internet sites and telephone advice centers to provide this type of support to their members. This level of enhanced communication and education is critical to achieve successful family-based care.

The new health care partnerships that use this approach have a responsibility to ensure that their home educators do not actually practice medicine. Even if electronic support is not yet available, manual self-care protocols with checks and balances can alert the patient and family members when they need to see someone skilled in disease treatment. One-on-one education shows families how to follow the protocol. When patients need a doctor immediately, they are directed by a triage protocol to go to the right professional. For the system to function effectively, the patient and the practice must cooperate. If the educator finds a problem, the protocol should recommend a same-day physician visit. Educators, nurses, allied health care professionals, physician assistants, and physicians should be focused on the goal of keeping the patient's care appropriate.

Reduced office visits, hospital stays, and pharmacy cost are just a few of the benefits of using family-focused care.

As shown in Figure 7.1, success in this model creates more reward, which stimulates more family-based care. This reinforcing system is critical to the new practice. High satisfaction and the perception of full access, reassure the practice that the reduced volume of care is not the result of rationing. The information support to track the success of this approach takes time to build into the practice infrastructure. At first, the information systems will need to be limited to the specific disease states for which the data show that self-care can save money as it manages disease. Once the new practice can succeed at this level of family-based cooperative care in partnership with all the other organizations across the continuum, the practice will have achieved the step needed to attempt a partnership with the community itself.

**Figure 7.1. Family-Based Care Reinforcing System.**

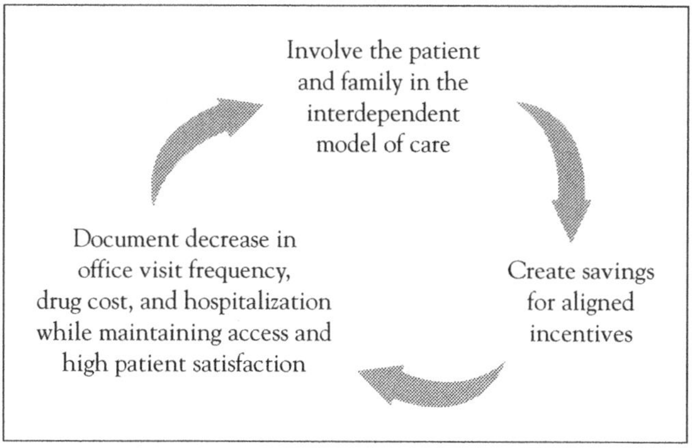

## Critical Elements

- Defining the family or support group for the patient.

- Designing an educational curriculum that changes physician and patient behavior.

- Understanding the culture/style of the key family members and the patient.

- Establishing a commitment to conduct patient/family education workshops.

- Tracking patient compliance in the home using mid-level providers.

- Developing a sequence of disease state triage steps from educator to specialist.

- Keeping a record of care provided and compliance achieved.

- Establishing a support system that answers families' questions outside of the office and triages for new medical problems.

- Analyzing outcomes obtained including cost accounting for ROI.

### NewMed Family Based Care

Karen was enjoying her new job. Her title was female family care coordinator, and like so many of the evolving allied health professional roles, her job description was in constant redesign.

Karen started as a RN before she became a diabetes educator, and then went on for her master's degree as a perinatal clinical specialist. This unique position with the NewMed group practice was the job she had been waiting for.

Karen approached the patient's house. Three men were talking in the front yard. She wondered whether one of them was Mr. Aguilar.

Gina was supposed to be at bed rest because of high blood pressure and a history of intrauterine growth retardation in her previous pregnancies. Karen hoped Gina was in bed. She rang the doorbell.

As Gina opened the door, Karen smiled and said, "What are you doing out of bed?"

"Oh, I've been down all day, but you know these kids, someone has to feed them."

Karen nodded.

"Where is Sergio?"

"Oh, he's over there."

Karen asked, "May I come in and take your blood pressure? I also need a urine sample."

"I know."

Karen paused. "This doesn't look like bed rest to me."

"No kidding!" Gina was getting irritated. "I've always been OK in the past."

Karen realized that Gina was the hub of the household and that no one else recognized the risk that she and the baby were in. "Where does your mom live?"

"Why do you want to know that?"

"Well, you need help Gina."

"I know, I know."

"Your pressure is up and you're getting protein in your urine. You know you could end up in the hospital again."

"I know."

"Would you be willing to attend some classes with your mom or your sister?"

Gina nodded, "I suppose."

Karen replied, "I could talk to them today if you feel it's OK."

Gina didn't respond.

"What is your mom's telephone number?"

Gina handed Karen a piece of paper with the number on it.

"It's either go to bed, Gina, or go to the hospital."

"I know," Gina replied.

"We need Sergio's help, too."

"He's outside."

"OK, you call your mom and I'll get Sergio."

Karen waved at Sergio, who was still talking to his neighbors. He came to the house slowly but his expression was one of concern.

Karen extended a hand, "Mr. Arguilar. It's a good thing you are at home right now, your wife is getting sick."

His concern deepened. "What is wrong?"

"Well the baby won't grow unless Gina can rest."

"It's a serious business, no?" Sergio replied, worried.

"Yes. I know she looks OK but her blood pressure is up. I need you to do a test on her urine every day, OK?"

"Sure it's OK, I can do it. I'll keep her down and I'll send the kids to her mother's. It's only a few weeks."

Karen nodded.

Karen knew that family care would be a challenge, but the neo-natal savings could be high if she succeeded. "I have videotapes in Spanish on your wife's condition. They will help both you and Gina's mother to see the real risk of Gina's condition. I will bring a portable VCR and TV here tomorrow. Can you get Gina's mother here?"

"Si."

She smiled and shook his hand. "Gracias!"

Karen went back to her car and opened her laptop to enter her notes.

"Imp. Chronic hypertension, One + urine protein, BP 135/80, thirty-two weeks gestation. Condition: Stable on bed rest. Plan: (1) Return in 24 hours for BP, urine/protein, and family education. (2) Husband and mother will provide support. (3) Children to stay at grandmother's house, all precautions understood; patient is assumed to be moder-ately compliant. (4) Follow-up with husband will be critical."

Karen walked back to the house to talk to Sergio.

"Two weeks—that's all we need."

This chapter has explored the often untapped potential of family involvement in the delivery of care as one of the key principles of the new practice of medicine. Details of the disease state manage-ment and the office practice structure needed to sustain this model are discussed in Chapters Ten and Eleven. As the patient, family, and the new practice partnership reach this level of patient-focused care, more opportunities open for partnership with the community. Chapter Eight describes the potential of the sixth and final dimen-sion, community partnerships.

# 8

# The Sixth Dimension
## *Partnering with the Community*

I n the last chapter, the organized involvement of families and support groups was demonstrated as a strategy to expand the potential of prevention and disease state management. In this chapter,
these principles, combined with the earlier dimensions, are expanded upon to include the scope of the entire community being
served. Until this step is achieved the new health partnerships fall
short of their ultimate potential. When all five of the preceding
dimensions are in place—integrated information exchange, aligned
incentives, clinical process improvement, high performance through
provider interdependence, and patient and family partnerships in
care—the sixth and final dimension, that of health care partnerships with the community can finally become a reality. The community actually helps the new practices become more successful at
managing disease, so both the community and the providers can
benefit economically.

## Community Partnerships

If the health care partnerships can decrease the number of patient
visits to the office or hospital while maintaining satisfaction and
access to patient care, the new practice of medicine will succeed. If
they succeed in decreasing the number of expensive drugs the patients need to take and the number of home visits they require,

there will be savings between what was budgeted for care and what the care actually cost. A portion of the savings is used to reward those who helped achieve the cost savings, but a part of the savings should be reinvested in the community. For instance, a practice could set up an account to reinvest savings to support specific projects in disease state management. These types of programs will also help practices and the community prepare for the future increases in population and aging.

A number of examples illustrating how community partnerships are being implemented throughout the United States are included in Chapter Thirteen. Although there are many challenges to implementing this model, a growing number of communities and practices are forging ahead. Before partnering can happen, the organizations within the new partnership must learn to cooperate rather than holding out for self-interest. When all parties in a community partnership are contributing, it creates a stronger, healthier community, increases interdependence of providers within the community as a whole, and increases likely savings in the cost of overall care.

What sets this model apart from the many other healthy-community efforts is that this approach is dependent on systems thinking and is driven by the benefits created from shared risk within an integrated health care partnership. The legalities of sharing financial risk and reward have been tested in courts state by state, and with the right type of partnership can be achieved. Community members must help remove legal barriers that might prevent shared information or aligned incentives for the clinical improvement described earlier. A good example is the provider-sponsored organization (PSO) in Albuquerque, New Mexico, where the state waived the restrictions that would have prevented a PSO from emerging.

Clinical process improvement (CPI) is another critical component in the partnering process. Measurement and reporting must prove that managing the disease and eliminating unnecessary care not only cuts costs, but also helps patients. The community partnership model also requires a cooperative focus on the family and a commitment to measure and monitor patient satisfaction and access. When both the medical community and the people served are sharing information and are mutually committed, the potential for success is great. Yet much of the current legislation actually inhibits community partnering.

Another challenge for physicians and the community is obtaining the overall data that show how widespread illness is and how effective care is becoming. For the first time, physicians can use community-wide data on specific diseases to identify solutions that have been overlooked because of the focus on the one-on-one patient encounter.

Once the practices and the public see data that describe the volume, type, and cost of care provided, insurance companies that independently gather information to set their cap limits safely in the profit column will lose their financial advantage over the new partnerships. Members of the community will be able to see the direct benefits that their efforts have on the community's health, regardless of the insurer, by accessing this data on the Internet. Until this level of community access to data can be established, the third-party payer is likely to retain its control in many communities.

Sharing summary reports of clinical outcomes community-wide is only possible when a strategic partnership of providers can be created. This point cannot be overemphasized. It is through a new health care partnership that communities can obtain new outcomes data to encourage and organize their volunteer efforts. In turn, these community groups can collect, analyze, and report accurate information at the point of care. The new medical practice can use the new data to incentivize those providing care. Because the community partnership is interdependent, both the community and the practices need to help each other get the data that prove they are succeeding. The data show the new partnership that they are succeeding in the specific areas of disease state management they have agreed to target for the community.

For example, teen pregnancy, teen violence, drug abuse, and gang crime are costly to every community. They devastate the families of those involved, the victims, and the entire community. Most providers never considered the real medical costs of these preventable conditions because the dollars spent in emergency room (ER) to care for the victims of these social ills could not be broken down. Information systems can now sort out the real costs required to treat the minds and bodies of these victims. And in the new practice, there is an incentive to track these costs. A community health project that takes on these issues encourages physicians to participate in reducing these social problems.

The community–physician partnership is discovering a new power to make an unprecedented impact on the community. In the new partnerships, abused women seen by physicians can be directed to safe houses and given counseling to break the cycle of abuse. When calling the police was the only option, physicians were often unable to help, and some women would stay in abusive situations for years. They would visit the ER regularly rather than risk sending an abusive husband to jail and ending what little support they had.

Patients with chronic illnesses can also benefit from community support. Many community public health programs have made nutritional counseling available for the indigent diabetic population, but because strong partnerships with physicians have not been created, or are without the right incentives, these services are dramatically underutilized (Close and others, 1992, p. 181).

Use of community volunteers to facilitate behavioral change in patients contributes a significant factor to ameliorating the severity of chronic conditions (Davis and others, 1998, p. 16). A physician clinic in Florida includes "lifestyle coaches" as part of their health care continuum. These individuals are employed by the clinic and provide education, feedback, and follow-up to patients. They target lifestyle issues such as nutrition, exercise, smoking cessation, and stress reduction (Collis, 1977, p. 19). This program promotes easy access for patient support and gives the physician more time to concentrate on truly sick patients. These same lifestyle coaches can magnify their own success by coaching other volunteers to become coaches themselves. In these new practices, physicians make public health efforts more successful by utilizing community services to improve medical outcomes.

## Defining the Community Partnership

The physician–community partnership is defined by its ability to think and act systematically by concentrating on a single goal and taking small, continuous steps toward its achievement. For example, the physician–community partnership might focus on management of childhood immunizations and use the office computer systems of small accountable groups of physicians to collect the data. This effort will not create short-term savings, but it helps build an information system that will provide information about the child as other problems occur. Physicians in the new practice see the need for the data link because it makes it more practical to track other clinical improvements.

Disease state management, such as decreasing pediatric asthma community-wide, certainly creates savings. By linking all of the new accountable practices across individual clinical improvement projects, the new practice can look at health systematically and community-wide. For instance, the community might provide education to families with children suffering from otitis media, or even sore throats. With that program in place the practice can track the occurrence and cost of treatment of these conditions one patient at a time. When this effort is conducted as a series of CPI studies, important clinical information is merged practice by practice to calculate the results and savings of the community-wide partnership.

## "Baby Your Baby"

In the past, many community efforts were impossible to maintain through the independent efforts of public health departments and others. The new practice of medicine will be able to drive those efforts successfully. An example of the old method helps make this point. In the 1980s, the Utah Governor's Council on Health and Fitness, along with a local TV station, the public health department, the Maternity and Infants Clinic at the University of Utah, and other community organizations from the Salt Lake City area, forged a comprehensive program called "Baby Your Baby." Their goal was to ensure that young and low-income pregnant women would receive appropriate education and prenatal care early enough to decrease low-for-gestational age birth weights and premature births substantially. The program gave $400 worth of coupons for food and other services to each woman who participated. If the patient saw a care provider early and frequently during her pregnancy, she received a coupon book. If she continued to go to the doctor, she received more coupons. "Baby Your Baby" was promoted by medical practices and by a large number of local businesses that donated these coupons for the advertising value. The program was a huge success and was picked up by many other states across the country.

Unfortunately, after two years, even though the original unpublished data showed that birth weights of babies had gone up and neonatal admissions in an indigent clinic population were reduced, the program's funding was cut due to faded enthusiasm. Because it was so expensive to track information in the 1980s, and the technological infrastructure was not in place, no effort was made to keep track of the savings. Because no one was rewarded for the success that was achieved, it was simply not sustained. As with so many similar, previous health efforts, the program directors decided to move on to another exciting project, and the benefits of their success with the "Baby Your Baby" program declined. If implemented across the United States, the potential savings from ongoing prevention of prematurity and decreased newborn ICU costs would be millions of dollars. Unfortunately, no one ever gathered the data to calculate return on the investment.

The new community partnerships will focus on this type of success instead of overlooking it. There are numerous examples of excellent public service efforts that lose funding after a short time. The projects save money, but no one tracks the savings and no one figures out who is benefitting from the savings. In most cases, these efforts are simply allowed to die out, but the new practice model can't afford to let that happen.

Physician-community partnerships measure success by the data, the improvement, the analysis, and the reward. Many community efforts fail because these dimensions are not in place, and the community organizations do not partner with accountable physician practices. Unless this happens, the communities will continue to fall far short of their health goals.

## Getting Started

A group of providers, a hospital, and a payer can build an infrastructure to implement the first five dimensions of the new practice. At this point they are able to form the community partnerships described here. The bigger the system, the harder it is to keep the strategy simple. Conversely, a single practice can actually partner with a community in a specific area. For example, Phoenix Pediatrics in Phoenix, Arizona engaged in a direct contract with the state to raise the level of care provided to multiply handicapped children in the city of Phoenix. This example is covered in detail in Chapter Eleven.

More commonly, the community partnership includes all of the patients and families of those seeking care from a single hospital or integrated system. A town or county can define the community. In areas that are small urban or rural, this community partnership is easy to conceptualize and define. Rural towns and small urban cities are creating integrated health care systems by combining several hospitals with less than 100 beds, home health care, and all the physicians who practice at those hospitals. This strategy not only helps the providers contract with insurers, it also provides the first step toward the new physician–community partnership.

In massive hospital-based integrated systems, it may be easier to limit the community to the patients in one hospital referral area. If multiple systems emerge in the same town (as is the case in most of urban America), the successful efforts of one new practice–community partnership will usually aid the community health efforts of the other hospitals in the referral area. If only one system adopts this approach, and the competing systems stay in the old practice of medicine, it only takes a few years for the new practice–community partnerships to gain market share over the competition (Robinson and Luft, 1985). Practices can publicize the fact that their patient population is simply healthier and their physicians are better, proven by the data showing that their patients need less care. Phoenix Pediatrics was almost too successful: They were audited to document that no fraud was present in their operations. The audit not only uncovered above-board operations but it also justified the practice's maintaining their level of reimbursement for all of the telephone triage and education that other practices didn't provide.

In Minneapolis and St. Paul, Minnesota, improvement data are released yearly by a large business coalition and have pushed competing integrated systems to accelerate disease state management. Allina Health Systems data on conditions such as congestive failure have shown steady improvement since the 1980s (Henry, 1998). In the Twin Cities, the public now expects improvement community-wide.

## A Step-Wise Approach

In the early stages of the new practice of medicine, the new health care partnership defines the critical health issues in the community that would decrease the real cost of medical care for the population covered by the new practice providers if these issues were well-managed. The group of patients surveyed can range from a single neighborhood to an entire state. For a successful physician–community partnership, the population must be defined and the key indicators of medical care (not all of the data) must be measured practice by practice throughout the entire target population. A small and manageable focus is obviously better than a large and all-inclusive one.

If several practices manage their own data collection within a single integrated partnership, they need data compatibility, communication systems, and information exchange to become truly integrated. This approach focuses on one disease at a time, so the data can be collected with personal computers (servers) or by using terminals connected to a central server over the Internet. This type of data integration is workable, as long as the collection and reporting systems are thought out in advance. The providers' level of commitment to sharing data determines how large a population can be addressed.

Once the physicians are committed to their role, the next step is to form volunteer subcommittees to outline the community interventions. For example, many states have recently begun to share statewide health data. Although still in the early stages, their first steps are to create a priority list of health issues (*Utah's Health*, 1996). This process can involve surveying a representative sample of all the health providers in the state or asking the public directly. The leaders in this process have recognized that success will not come from the public health department alone or any other single system, but from a clear plan for improvement that affects everyone.

### Focus Down

A good strategy for partnerships is to target one health issue and widely manage the disease state. This also benefits the hospital and physicians. If the practices are motivated to implement the single improvement, and summary reports of their efforts are linked together across the Internet, the public impact can be documented in less than a year. A successful effort depends on the ability of the community to encourage and coordinate the efforts of the practicing physicians. If the community can reward small, accountable groups of physicians for being agents of change and physicians continue to compete with each other to be the best, the improvement effort will be dramatically accelerated.

The best course for small states or larger cities is to pick a single health issue like pediatric asthma and assist individual practices with managing this disease. HMOs will provide an incentive for successful practices to reap the economic rewards while the community gains the benefit of better health. The community can focus on additional health issues once the first success is achieved.

The physician–community partnership must choose a disease that is preventable or at least manageable, such as pneumonia or congestive heart failure. By building on one success after another, true health care reform can be achieved. Unfortunately, this type of strategic planning and information sharing at the state level is still rare. This is largely due to the fact that only a few insurance companies are developing plans to share data. These old patterns of thinking are based on distrust and are slowing community efforts to make the new practice of medicine a statewide goal.

The success of the new practice requires a community-by-community approach within each state or city. State and federal governments need to make a commitment to promote this model of care, or at least not stand in its way because of political self-interest. Until then, efforts are best focused on smaller patient populations that can be managed by the new health care partnerships.

### Begin the Education

More education and training are needed to improve the community's understanding of key health issues. Data are already being used to teach the right lessons to the right people in many communities. Seeing data that prove successful results have been achieved by volunteer community members increases the community's enthusiasm to keep helping. This means that clear and frequent reports need to become a part of the community partnership strategy to keep this reinforcing loop moving. The reward of seeing the effect of one's own work through data may be the most important driving force behind genuine health care reform at the community level. For example, the impact of teen pregnancy mentors in a Detroit project to educate single adolescents as a method to lower pregnancy rates was publicized. The visible success immediately increased the number of volunteers as the pregnancy rate continued to decline (Carlson, 1994, p. 67). If the data are not reassuring, individuals can also stop efforts that are not working. Either way, both the community and the new practices benefit by sharing data.

## Critical Elements

- Defining the community as a population.
- Finding out what community support could help specific patients.
- Eliciting the support of community volunteers.
- Implementing an improvement strategy by using CPI.
- Keeping the effort simple and focused.
- Agreeing to manage a single disease.
- Tracking clinical indicators at the practice level.
- Keeping data compatible across the system.
- Tracking population statistics one practice at a time.
- Using the data to inspire the community to keep helping.
- Creating a payer contract to share risk and reward.
- Planning for reward and reinvestment.
- Reinvesting in the community support.

### The Community and NewMed Celebrate

The celebration had only been under way a few hours when Bill looked back at the other physicians and the administrators who were serving as the hosts to hundreds of community members gathered in the park.

Bill turned to Kenny, "You know this partnership actually works because of those volunteers. This event is the culmination of a five-year effort to reach the elderly and the troubled youth in the poorest sections of town."

"Absolutely, these are the people who succeeded. This is really their celebration."

"Look at these people. The majority is gray or balding, but some are gang kids wearing their gang colors. The one common denominator is that they are all smiling."

"I know, it's great. The award ceremony is certainly being well attended. And look, isn't that Channel 5 news?"

"It is Kenny, now that's justice! The media are finally picking this up."

"Well why not? Pulmonary disease and heart disease have each been cut by a third in the elderly population. That's awesome."

"I don't know, the 40 percent reduction in neonatal admissions of Medicaid babies is what impresses me."

"Yes, it's odd how all of this has evolved. We started training volunteers in our free HMO clinic as part of the system commitment to reinvest some of the clinical savings back into the community. And then we were able to use the same volunteers as patient partners to make home and school visits that affected our other patients."

Bill smiled. "Yes, it's all working out very well."

"You know it's not the awards that are important. It's that the public's health status has actually been improved. The frequency of disease decreased because the physicians and the community decided to make it a common goal."

Bill nodded. He was proud that NewMed was the best of the best. He thought about the old days and how Kenny had really been able to see the future. Kenny knew that these organizations could reach the same levels of cooperation that his PAQ helped to pioneer.

"I think we are safe for a few years, Kenny, but what if we ever stop cooperating?"

"Good point, I guess we can't stop."

Kenny and Bill both smiled and clapped as the award ceremony began.

This chapter has emphasized the importance of maintaining a community focus as continuous improvement of clinical care is proven to create a healthier population. The infrastructure needed to support communication and information exchange within this new practice of medicine at the system partnership level will be discussed in Chapter Nine. Chapter Nine also outlines the support needed to accelerate the implementation of the learning within the six dimensions of the new practice of medicine. The principles in Chapter Nine are then reinforced in Chapter Ten, which details methods to focus on disease state management as the building blocks for change. Chapter Eleven goes on to explain the physician's role within practices accountable for quality (PAQ). The success of the PAQ strategy serves as the backbone of the new practice partnerships as they strive to improve the health of the community they serve.

# 9

# Building an Infrastructure for Learning

The last six chapters explored the major principles at work within the transformation of medical care delivery. In this chapter, these theories are applied as an organizational infrastructure capable of supporting physician change. The purpose, layout, project design, and general organization of an office to facilitate communication and information exchange are described. The chapter also focuses on use of an assessment to guide the development of the office based on financial forecasts and ongoing evaluation of operations. Finally, a method to establish this office and overcome the challenges of operating it is offered.

Unlike the old medical environment, the new practice of medicine must nurture interdependency, accountability, learning, and communication. A cornerstone of the new practice is to utilize data, but not everything that the data show will be reassuring. If problems are exposed, the physicians may develop defensive behavior. Some physicians may fear that they will be embarrassed or lose prestige. Because the public now has the ability to compare physician data, many health care professionals feel as if they are in a win-lose situation (Carpenter, Swerdlow, and Fear, 1997, p. 388).

The emerging integrated partnerships need to ensure that their physicians win in these data comparisons. To do this, a new level of trust and an internal commitment to helping the physician practices change are needed. These practices need education and technical support to be able to place themselves in the top 50 percent prior to outside comparisons. That means that internal confidential comparisons must be made to guide improvements before the outcome comparisons are made public. Fear and resistance are a natural part of any major organizational change, but professional partnerships using data, constant communication, shared risk, and joint accountability driven by systems thinking can support the new practice through the change. Partners must develop a step-by-step organizational redesign or reinvention of themselves within the new health care environment. A responsive organizational structure can overcome resistance and sustain needed changes.

The new partnership needs an office that acts as a hub for change based on facts. For descriptive purposes here, we'll call it the clinical information management and communication office, or CIMCO. CIMCO is not the information systems (IS) department of a hospital, though it may depend on IS support. CIMCO is the hub for continuous learning within the partnership itself, dedicated to the sole purpose of communicating the facts needed to operationalize the strategy for the new practice of medicine. Good clinical judgments, acts, and controlled access to the right data support CIMCO. CIMCO is the brain of the new partnership, signaling and stimulating the many professional groups that make up the nervous system of the new practice partnerships. What is more important, CIMCO provides direction for education, feedback, reward, and new clinical performance. This model uses systems thinking and a communication strategy that creates discrete data messages that are clean and accurate. CIMCO sends clear messages back to the response area, that is, any location where care is provided. CIMCO continuously adds new knowledge based on real experience.

CIMCO implements the specific data management and coordination steps needed by the new practice of medicine. By using fact-based clinical information to answer specific questions of importance to physicians, CIMCO establishes feedback through clear regular reports. If this critical level of communication is not accomplished, the result is "information overload" that directs the physicians in large health care systems in nonproductive or even harmful ways. In a nutshell, the goal of CIMCO is to generate specific computerized decision support systems to accelerate the implementation of strategies for quality improvement and disease state management. CIMCO also accounts for the financial impact throughout the partnership. Because CIMCO fills so many critical functions, the partnership should create a business plan for CIMCO as though it were a business within the system that guides the partnership. Prior to this first step, the partnership must describe the purpose of building a support structure for communication and information exchange.

## The Purpose of CIMCO

CIMCO's primary purpose is to communicate new information in a way that motivates and supports physicians and management as they implement positive change. CIMCO's findings are used for education and incentives that encourage new physician behavior. The goal is to foster a more integrated and interdependent model of care that can also prove that health is improving. With data, CIMCO builds needed trust between the physicians and managers of the many organizations that make up the new partnerships. CIMCO uses the data to improve clinical decision making and to reinforce new physician behavior. The CIMCO team coordinates the data to design, develop, and implement new clinical knowledge.

More important, they counter physicians' defensiveness with high-level communication and tailored education based on the data. Replacing defensive reasoning with productive fact-based reasoning results in the implementation of care improvements that ensure the success of physicians and the partnership. CIMCO strategies are developed from sound business principles and the growing body of scientifically valid research on clinical improvement, structures for disease state management, and organizational learning. The strategies are also culled from practice assessments conducted by the physicians themselves. CIMCO reports whatever data the physicians have defined as a valid indicator of change. The results of clinical process improvement (CPI) data, organizational assessments, practice analysis, and physician attitude surveys all clarify what challenges professionals face, as well as what they value. This information can be used to design specific education and decision support that is clearly valuable to the particular groups of physicians who are trying to change.

Physicians can direct their own change process with this type of grassroots personalized clinical data, integrated with the education and communication strategies described here. CIMCO provides the support by organizing improvements in physician practice that draw on CPI and computerized technical supports (as reviewed in Chapter Five). Next, this improvement approach is linked to physician high-performance training (as described in Chapter Six). CIMCO's goals are designed to ensure the highest possible quality of care, the lowest necessary cost and liability risk, and the least restriction on physician decision making. These goals must all be accomplished without harming the physician-patient relationship. Organizations that have successfully met these goals have focused on the core professional values of the physicians and other health care providers and on communicating specific facts that overcome resistance to change.

CIMCO is also responsible for establishing the technical link between the executive leadership of the system and the clinical and management staff. This link is created and maintained through clear, focused reporting and fact-based communication. This critical function of tracking, reporting, communication, and education is needed to ensure rapid and sound decision making at the point of care. Many other top-down approaches have failed because of physicians' resistance and a lack of commitment. This information link also uses ongoing feedback (reports) to reassure physicians as they attempt to share new clinical roles with many new providers. Without a CIMCO support strategy, new partnerships will inevitably fail to overcome internal resistance. Transformation can only occur when physicians are provided with the data that will help them achieve what they value.

For example, IHC's Institute for Health Care Delivery Research assists its hospitals in analyzing and organizing physician practice patterns into feedback reports that are given to the physicians one diagnosis at a time. The IHC Institute brings potential direction and assistance to the changes from which all IHC facilities could benefit. With the addition of a behavioral change focus and aligned incentives, CIMCO completes this type of approach by establishing a clear connection between the practicing physician's willingness to experiment in improvement and the reward that sustains motivation. This combination dramatically accelerates learning.

## Critical Elements of CIMCO

The success of any institute or office that must coordinate change lies in its ability to accelerate implementation of new processes. To help key partners work together and get results a basic structure to guide operations is needed.

### The Layout of the Office

The initial structure for CIMCO should include an operating plan, budget, and an outline of the financial and human resources requirements for supporting the operation of the office. Next, the partnership should perform an evaluation of the staffing requirements, personnel time, communication processes, and coordination strategies.

Individuals who are most likely to benefit from a fully operational CIMCO should be identified. These individuals will become the champions and leaders of CIMCO. Clinical department heads, as well as informed physician leaders, are then brought together with quality and operational managers. When organized, this group will lead the communication and information exchange process.

The scope of work for this group includes the following responsibilities:

- Establishing an operational interface for CIMCO within the system

- Establishing a feedback structure for reward, recognition, and communication to drive improvement

- Evaluating management and staffing considerations

- Analyzing funding and budgetary issues

- Identifying resources necessary to launch the office and manage change

- Carrying out the clinical and financial improvement analysis and reporting on physician effectiveness and simple improvement projects

- Facilitating physician peer education and ongoing communication of success

### Staffing CIMCO

CIMCO should be staffed in a stepwise manner, that is, adding staff only as they are needed to carry out specific agendas. Initially, the staff might include only a special projects coordinator and an administrator. Later, a full-time financial analyst may be needed. Eventually, most offices will need at least two data analysts and at least two part-time physicians passionate about CPI and clinical effectiveness. Staff members must be able to use software applications that draw on key variables being used throughout the system to create selective reports. New reporting and communication of facts are not optional. Personnel must learn to use statistical display software or SAGE™ type reporting tools to create nearly real-time graphics and results needed for physician peer discussion.

The temptation is to try to run this office with one or two employees as an adjunct to their regular job duties. This approach is doomed from the start. Most organizations have failed to motivate physician change because of a slow start and poor quality results. An ineffective CIMCO is possibly the biggest obstacle an integrated system can face as it attempts to accelerate the physician partnerships needed for transformation.

## Project Design and Information Management

Although strategic planning and operationalizing services can begin immediately, it will take a few months to complete a retrospective assessment of data needed to establish benchmarks and to agree on the first targeted improvement projects. Retrospective data can clarify current care processes, potential improvements, and savings that can be achieved through intervention strategies in each of the study variables selected. Data sources often include chart review, discharge data, pharmacy data, and financial and utilization data. If a retrospective look at the data is not feasible, it is possible to start the same type of data collection immediately and view it as a baseline after six months of collection.

Details of CPI and layout were included in Chapter Five and a model of disease state management (DSM) is included in the next chapter. In general, scope of work for an organized improvement project includes the following critical elements, often accomplished in the following order:

1. Determining potential clinical outcomes

2. Validating data sources

3. Assessing computerized information capabilities

4. Analyzing current data systems

5. Establishing clinical improvement tracking systems

6. Collecting retrospective data for initial projects

7. Identifying prospective data collection criteria

8. Analyzing clinical data of the improvement effort

9. Managing knowledge service alerts and knowledge bases

10. Establishing educational curriculums

11. Managing implementation of change

12. Rewarding those who are successful

This fundamental model provides the structure to launch the work of CIMCO.

### Organization of the Clinical Data Office

The structure of CIMCO includes four fundamental operating divisions under the guidance of a steering committee: CPI design and development, CPI implementation and redesign, information management, and education and communication (see Figure 9.1). Each division has a specific focus and is responsible for implementing specific projects that make up their division's work tasks. They are also interdependent, an interdependence facilitated by sharing data reports and by continuous dialogue among personnel. As CIMCO grows, personnel often work in more than one of these four divisions.

These four operating divisions focus on clinical improvement, coordinated data collection and measurement, designing dynamic practice guidelines, communicating success, and creating training programs. CIMCO's work accelerates and sustains the gains from revenue generation and documented improvements in clinical outcomes. CIMCO accounts for impact, reward, and reinvestment. The steering committee retains the ultimate authority for how savings are managed according to the contracted agreements they manage. These contracted agreements are negotiated by the top executive leadership within the partnership organizations. The formulas for analyzing and reporting results are based upon business formulas designed to achieve and maintain visible fairness.

**Figure 9.1. The Clinical Data Office Organizational Model.**

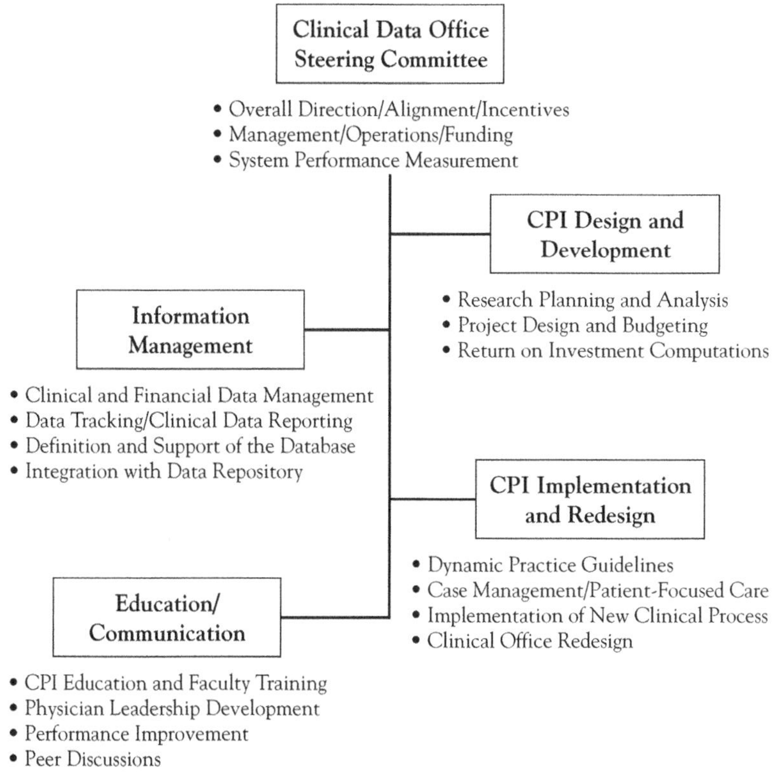

```
            ┌─────────────────────────┐
            │   Clinical Data Office  │
            │   Steering Committee    │
            └─────────────────────────┘
```

• Overall Direction/Alignment/Incentives
• Management/Operations/Funding
• System Performance Measurement

```
                          ┌─────────────────────┐
                          │   CPI Design and    │
                          │    Development      │
                          └─────────────────────┘
```

                          • Research Planning and Analysis
                          • Project Design and Budgeting
                          • Return on Investment Computations

```
  ┌─────────────────────┐
  │     Information     │
  │     Management      │
  └─────────────────────┘
```

• Clinical and Financial Data Management
• Data Tracking/Clinical Data Reporting
• Definition and Support of the Database
• Integration with Data Repository

```
                          ┌─────────────────────────┐
                          │  CPI Implementation     │
                          │     and Redesign        │
                          └─────────────────────────┘
```

                          • Dynamic Practice Guidelines
                          • Case Management/Patient-Focused Care
                          • Implementation of New Clinical Process
                          • Clinical Office Redesign

```
  ┌─────────────────────┐
  │     Education/      │
  │    Communication    │
  └─────────────────────┘
```

• CPI Education and Faculty Training
• Physician Leadership Development
• Performance Improvement
• Peer Discussions

## Creating an Operational Plan

The success or failure of any new organizational structure depends on an overall plan and a strong operational design. This design starts with a reporting blueprint that will be used later to tailor an implementation assessment and plan. Before the implementation steps can be designed and put in place, an overall plan must be constructed. It should include the following components:

- Physician/executive commitment and leadership

- Financial/clinical information support that is reliable and timely

- Expertise to design clinical improvements and guide the implementation process

- A communication strategy that can dynamically tailor reports of success to specific groups

Identifying people and processes necessary for the implementation of improvement projects is one of the early responsibilities of the steering committee. Once this initial targeting step is accomplished, it becomes possible for the committee to evaluate which dynamic practice guidelines and clinical redesign models are likely to be acceptable to the interdependent professional groups delivering care.

Eventually, all of the contemplated change will be integrated into a system of *knowledge alerts*. These knowledge alerts link the correct information with providers across the continuum of care. First, the partnership must concentrate on simple projects with simple reports at the local level to successfully launch CIMCO.

Additional individuals who will be involved in the CIMCO management and operational structure are selected on a project basis by the steering committee. Individuals with experience in research design and implementation of clinical improvements can be recruited from internal physician leadership and information resources throughout the partnership organizations. The steering committee's selection is based on the individual's willingness and ability to participate in protocol development, therapy selection, knowledge engineering, change management, and data reporting. The CIMCO leadership will need to grow as complexity increases, so it is best to start small but budget for rapid growth.

## Data Management

It is helpful to include an organization that is sophisticated and large enough to have an IS department. This may be a hospital, MSO, or even an insurance company, but it must be willing to enter into an open partnership dedicated to the rigorous management of data. CIMCO needs data support to achieve accessible, reliable, and timely communication of data reports. By adding this reporting service to the large information support structures, data management can quickly be applied to research and financial analysis. Because CIMCO needs to report on consistent rapid success, they should have the highest priority when requesting the packaging of specific data from information services. The highest priority requests made by CIMCO to IS will reflect the strategy of top management and physician leadership. For instance, the strategy may focus on critical results of office practice improvements, disease state management, or larger CPI projects. Usually, these projects will rely on widespread computer-aided decision making. For example, a pharmacy utilization improvement may require IS to retool the pharmacy database to include reminders. Because these decisions have major cost considerations, high-ranking representatives from all IS departments are essential members of the CIMCO steering committee.

## Funding

It is important to prove that CIMCO will actually provide revenues sufficient to cover the first or second year's start-up costs. The operating capital needed for rewarding new behavior, reporting on results, and launching subsequent studies must be provided even though the return might be delayed. Sufficient funding for the requisite early work needs to be budgeted and firmly committed to. For example, CIMCO can project an estimate of savings if 100 percent of the clinical improvement and disease state management goals are achieved. This figure is equal to 100 percent of the achievable return on investment. The actual data is then compared to this figure to give a progress report. Success is reported as a percentage of achievable return on investment. The expenses are also tracked as a percentage of what is projected. Partnerships find that costs and savings against projections can be tracked in monthly reports. These data are then used to trend further success or failure.

## The CIMCO Implementation Assessment

Once the purpose of the CIMCO office is clear and a structural plan of operation is in place, an assessment should be conducted to link the implementation of change to the strategic plan of the new health care partnership. The first step is to list clinical outcomes that could be improved throughout the system by instituting standardized protocols and processes to support clinical decision making. These improvements must lead to reduced costs of clinical care. After these projects are prioritized, a few targets are decided on. The second step is to outline a feasibility plan to establish shared risk or gain sharing as a reward for each involved physician's success at improvement. The feasibility worksheet in Chapter Five describes the potential for savings.

For example, some systems have found that the easiest way to reward the physician is to pay them 25 percent of what the feasibility forecast projects will be returned after the cost of the project is subtracted from the savings. This can be applied as an hourly consulting fee paid to cover the time physicians spend on the actual improvement project, CIMCO meetings, education, and protocol development. This incentive makes it more likely that they will be willing to spend time away from their practices. Adding bonuses for timely completion of the project or for achieving specific clinical outcomes is more complex and always requires legal advice, but the results are worth the effort.

## Focusing the Forecasts

Forecasts are necessary to account for substantial and immediate real dollar savings based on a wide variety of payer contracts. As a result, it is important to assess the information links between the specific clinical improvements and financial results. If absent, information links will need to be put in place so that they aid in the reporting of success. Executive support for these new information links must also be assessed. If executives are not committed, it is pointless to move on.

A means of documenting that the incentives from the savings are fairly and reliably distributed according to partnership agreements is another necessity.

The partnership should agree on the amount of sustained, continuous return on investment required to drive the new practice in the future and outline their commitment in writing as a clear framework for change. An assessment can determine where the enhanced management of acute and chronic illness across the continuum of care will create needed savings. The organizations within the new partnership should try to imagine where their health care delivery services will be in the next five years. Knowledge engineering and specific reporting will probably be a requirement to support clinical improvement efforts. But more important, a plan to achieve a return on investment after specific landmarks are reached should lead the partnership to a completely redesigned approach to care. This plan will make it important to understand how information systems and Internet server technology can support analysis and rapid communication. At the same time new relationships will need to be evaluated according to the agreed upon scope of change. Forecasting can be used to explore all these issues and track them against expectations.

To reach this level of preparation, a flexible and responsive leader and a management infrastructure that can adapt to the use of new data (feedback) are required. A management assessment will predict the likelihood of CIMCO being aligned with the strategic plan of the partnership organizations. There must be alignment if CIMCO is to take on real responsibility. The forecasts must include a budget directed toward the redesign described here, or implementation of rapid dynamic change is unlikely.

### Evaluating Operations

Best-care standards in one area are defined by careful observation of actual practice. While one interdependent practice is improving, new ideas are naturally shared with other practices. This improvement method is based on collaboration and cooperation and driven by compelling data and sound clinical information. Increased multidisciplinary clinical team cooperation and high performance will also require new operational planning and support. New team training should be implemented that will result in physicians' expanding their use of interdependent delivery models in partnership with ancillary providers. Physicians need cross-education so they can think as a cooperative group. CIMCO will obviously need a new approach to communication and education to achieve the changes outlined.

The CIMCO assessment must detail these operational challenges and demonstrate a reasonable likelihood that this level of organizational change is feasible. For example, an operational plan that includes the additional burden of tasks usually managed by IS, quality assurance (QA), or credentialing will have problems. Confidentiality and accountability issues in QA and credentialing are strict and very different from the goals of an improvement research focus. Because of the traditionally punitive use of data that evolved under QA, the CIMCO approach must stay separate to reinforce cooperation and trust.

As a final step, an assessment of physician attitudes regarding the use of data is used to track the progress of improvement and reward strategies managed within CIMCO.

## Establishing CIMCO

After reviewing the assessment results, many partnerships are overwhelmed by all the steps necessary for CIMCO to achieve total success. Keep in mind that only a few steps are needed to get CIMCO started. Planning a development sequence is recommended to ensure that each step paves the way for the next. Caution should temper excess enthusiasm. Some will try to implement all these principles at once overwhelming the staff. A CIMCO plan should be implemented slowly over the course of a year. A balanced approach to expansion is needed for the support of the partnership.

### Understanding the Educational Challenge

For information selection, collection, and analysis to be useful, early professional education must be conducted. The educational component is focused on the actual delivery of care via an experience-based curriculum to educate physicians whose training did not include business principles. The skills of managing disease states or using population-based data to define best practice must also be included. The CPI model described in Chapter Five can be used to organize new expectations for physicians to deliver new, but established, best-care practices. The goal of CIMCO is to help physicians learn from the results. This can be facilitated by teaching financial analysis and business accounting principles. The goal is to create a link between finance and clinical outcome. Though the lessons will vary, critical factors will always include teaching the concepts of CPI as an influence on the business principles of the system.

CIMCO's need for data is dependent on the partnership's business contracts, which set physicians' expectations. An incentive plan defines the reports that will motivate the physicians as improvements are implemented. Physicians should be prepared for the possibility that real costs will be higher than budgeted costs. There also needs to be a clear plan for distributing any dollar savings that physicians achieve. For this to occur, physicians should know how to use a clear and open accounting method to demonstrate how the interdependent parts of the new practice either created the opportunity for reward or contributed to risk. Without this step in information management, parts of the system are likely to be inappropriately rewarded while others are ignored. The inability to allocate resources fairly and physicians' lack of business knowledge have led to the distrust that many physicians and hospitals have come to expect.

Because CIMCO's purpose is the coordination of facts to accelerate change, CIMCO should create an environment that helps physicians learn from themselves as they respond to market forces under managed care. Because of the expectation to change focus constantly and rapidly, CIMCO must plan to continuously manage conflict resolution, joint decision making, and accountability. Cooperation is the source of real-time learning driven by facts and sharing risk and reward, as opposed to the old medicine's focus on managing time and working harder. CIMCO supports doing only what is needed for the well-being of the patient instead of doing as much as can be done as quickly as possible.

The educational job of CIMCO is very strict. It is responsible to educate physicians specifically while integrating the care they deliver within the system. CIMCO analyzes and communicates new knowledge based on specific data to particular groups of physicians, thereby directing the next specific educational efforts. Because CIMCO establishes clear channels of accountability and helps the physicians understand the data, those who decide where to sacrifice and where to give rewards turn to CIMCO for direction. Providers use CIMCO to see an accounting of how well their expectations were fulfilled. From clerical help to the top management, CIMCO operations are based on facts, communication, and accountability.

### The Steering Committee

A CIMCO steering committee uses the data generated within the overall integrated delivery system to direct CIMCO operations, and

CIMCO uses data to move the system toward success. The top executive leadership of the integrated partnership directs the CIMCO steering committee. This ensures clear direction. It also clarifies top management's true intentions to the entire system. The steering committee must act quickly on the expectations of the partnership leaders. From the committee flows the implementation effort, where plans are carried out, modified, or abandoned—all of which is visible to the entire system.

CIMCO data create trust by defining visible fairness through the open use of information to achieve improvement and reward. This data analysis affects education and redesign. CIMCO data can also expose the failure to implement best intentions. This failure is often an unexpected result of early change efforts. For example, a failed effort to achieve the stated milestones for improvement and savings can lead to blame. The failure to succeed needs to be anticipated and the results seen as an opportunity to rebuild in order to succeed next time. Such a failure should be followed with a formal peer discussion and a serious effort to help the individuals in the project succeed. The steering committee may request a redesign of a major part of the system to ensure such a success. If the failure is ignored and there is no follow-up, this will be a major setback in the effort to build physician trust.

Because the strength of CIMCO is measured by accountability, the steering committee must select projects carefully. Efforts that have succeeded elsewhere can be implemented by CIMCO. Systematic implementation of known CPI support measures from Chapter Five can be helpful in this situation. Projects should be completed according to a strict timeline and rewards given immediately thereafter. These guiding principles of the success of CIMCO are the mission of the steering committee.

The steering committee faces a difficult challenge when approving the effective use of selected, high-priority information. Sabotage of the work in midstream, or even worse—falsifying or selectively omitting data—is possible. If CIMCO cannot maintain high-level self-scrutiny, it runs the risk of being accused of wrongdoing, a serious threat to trust within the system. CIMCO cannot measure everything, so the steering committee must set a clear and narrow focus. If a request is too broad or general in nature, the CIMCO steering committee refers it to IS.

CIMCO is committed to focused systems thinking that uses business computations, clinical analysis, cooperation, and clear reports of results. All of this work is confidential and is maintained within a management structure maintaining the highest level of integrity. This unique office maintains the reports that build trust through visible fairness. CIMCO also determines which summary data should remain accessible as long as proper precautions and clearances are achieved. The steering committee must handle this responsibility wisely. Open review of successful summary data is critical, but at the same time confidentiality must be maintained on an individual level. The committee sets the guidelines for access to data through executive input from all the partnership organizations. Those eligible to see the graphic display of population summary data should include anyone involved in its collection or anyone internal to the system who could be affected by the success or failure of a given study. Data on individual providers is only revealed to the providers themselves. In some systems, these reports are only accessible with a personal access code and must be viewed on a personal computer. This prevents a written report from getting into the wrong hands. This trust-building responsibility of the steering committee cannot be overemphasized. CIMCO must retain openness while protecting the confidentiality of individual physicians.

### Overcoming the Challenges of Operation

Extracting needed data out of chaos is a major operation of CIMCO. The information captured needs to be practically measurable, important, and relevant to a specific group of providers who want to change care. CIMCO's operations create focus through a utility matrix that scores priority (see Table 9.1). This matrix lists possible projects in a column; then across the top of the page it lists success criteria such as cost, clinical relevance, etc. Point values for low and high subjective, but informed, impressions are then assigned to issues. For example, high volume might get a three and low volume receive a one. Other categories are clinical importance, fixed payer margin, a physician champion, known method for improvement, and information availability. The high-scoring project will have the highest sum of the points from the success criteria. This mechanical approach can set the priorities for an entire system in a matter of hours.

A major operational task is coordination of new information and communication interfaces between providers. Communication of information clearly influences costs. The individual needs of each accountable practice cannot be ignored by CIMCO, even if there

**Table 9.1. Utility Matrix.**

|  | Quality | Finance | External Customers | Operational Feasibility | Total |
|---|---|---|---|---|---|
| Coronary bypass | 3.0 | 3.0 | 2.0 | 2.7 | 2.7 |
| Major joints | 2.7 | 3.0 | 2.5 | 2.3 | 2.6 |
| ICU | 3.0 | 3.0 | 2.2 | 2.3 | 2.6 |
| Cardiac valve proc. | 2.7 | 3.0 | 2.0 | 2.7 | 2.6 |
| Pneumonia | 2.7 | 3.0 | 2.5 | 2.0 | 2.5 |
| Myocardial infarct | 2.3 | 3.0 | 2.5 | 2.0 | 2.5 |
| Adverse drug events | 2.7 | 2.5 | 2.0 | 2.3 | 2.4 |
| Pressure sores | 2.3 | 2.5 | 2.0 | 2.0 | 2.2 |
| Major bowel proc. | 2.0 | 3.0 | 2.0 | 1.7 | 2.2 |
| Rehabilitation | 1.7 | 3.0 | 2.0 | 2.0 | 2.2 |
| Deep venous thromb. | 2.3 | 2.5 | 2.0 | 1.7 | 2.1 |
| Deep P.O. wound inf. | 2.0 | 2.0 | 1.5 | 2.7 | 2.0 |
| CHF | 2.0 | 3.0 | 1.5 | 1.7 | 2.0 |
| Tracheotomy | 1.3 | 3.0 | 2.0 | 1.0 | 1.8 |
| Women's services | 1.7 | 0.0 | 3.0 | 2.3 | 1.8 |
| Chest pain | 2.7 | 0.0 | 1.0 | 2.0 | 1.4 |

Reproduced courtesy of Intermountain Health Care.

is conflict. Resistance to change is predictable and can be managed with organized reporting that is supported by dialogue and constant communication. CIMCO staff must help the clinical groups involved give up old methods and measures that do not contribute to positive change.

CIMCO creates new interfaces between previously divergent groups, one disease at a time. As care moves out of the hospital, CIMCO must create a new focus to build data interfaces that allow for data collection and transfer to the CIMCO reporting tools. These new connections eventually will include the physician practices and home health care. The outpatient management of disease will eventually be linked to a variety of community interfaces. This will also be part of CIMCO's challenge, but practice interfaces come first. For example, a business that has added health care personnel and computerized patient education on site can be a formal part of a strategy for disease state management. In this case, CIMCO can build the data link between the business and the physician practices only if the physician office is already connected to CIMCO. At this level of information exchange the impact on the business's employees can be compared to other patient populations.

Interfacing operationally with complex organizations dedicated to their own self-interest makes a common commitment and accountability within any integrated system difficult. Each individual group within the partnership must be technically linked to the CIMCO's operational plan through feedback of data. CIMCO creates and shares key data reports that encourage cooperation, process improvement, and system-wide integration. These reports are timely and well-documented, and they clarify any possible rewards. CIMCO staff must foster a willingness to share reports within each of the many groups and organizations that make up the partnership. Key individuals are responsible as liaisons, partners, educators, and enablers, in addition to their usual roles. CIMCO provides these new leaders with the means to communicate via common tools, resources, and education. This level of interaction and cooperation is possible because CIMCO stays focused on one complete set of cause-and-effect system relationships while tracking the flow of care in a defined and accountable group one disease state at a time. Because the outside pressures on the health systems are not allowed to overwhelm CIMCO, it works on individual projects until they are completed, then moves on to the next project. The cumulative impact of these projects will bring about the success that many integrated systems have thought to be impossible.

### Finding a Context for Work

CIMCO sets the course for change, provides education, establishes the model of project implementation, and provides feedback to those who provide care. All these functions must be placed in context with the marketplace forces that define reimbursement and market share. Maintaining provider relationships and communicating discouraging shifts in the very real payer environment will be one of the major challenges of this office. As a result, the partnership should plan on abandoning old priorities on a regular basis and communicating new data management strategies that are central to success.

### Giving Physicians What They Value

Resolving the tension created when physicians feel that the system won't let them do what they value professionally is a critical task of the office. This gap between what physicians value and what they believe they can do within the system is a major reason that physicians are resisting change. The new practice aligns what physicians value and what they can actually accomplish and holds that up as a guide for all that follows. A national survey entitled *Integrated Medical Partnerships Aligned for Quality* (IMPAQ) is being conducted in association with VHA, Inc.'s Physician Leadership Program, which started in 1996 (Prather and others, 1999). The survey contains questions designed to clarify what physicians want out of practice. A rating scale was used to analyze what physicians value as they move into a more managed and more accountable health care environment. These results were then contrasted to the same rating scale evaluating what the physicians felt they were actually doing.

Seeing what physicians believe reality to be as opposed to what they want has created a critical guide for education. The physicians outlined action steps to help them get what they want, and the subsequent educational design followed the physicians' lead. The IMPAQ data clearly showed that a new level of cooperation between physician groups is highly valued but not generally in place. It also pointed to a nationwide conflict of values between specialists and primary care providers. Both sides feel the other group is invading their professional turf, even though they have no facts to verify these assumptions. Physicians value having improvement data, but in most cases believe it is not accessible.

For the purposes of this discussion, the central finding of the survey was the very high value that physicians placed on sharing in the savings that they create as they help improve care. Although the value for participating in shared risk contracts is very high, most physicians feel helpless to achieve this opportunity. Integrated systems across the country are making a major mistake by ignoring physicians' deep unrest from the opinion that they are being treated unfairly. CIMCO responds to this type of unrest with a clear plan and creates reports that use the partnership's business logic to illustrate how physicians are succeeding in gain-sharing arrangements. (This is further explained in Chapter Three, Figure 3.2.)

**Supporting Physician Change**

CIMCO performs the analysis and reports the results that can potentially close the gaps between what physicians value and what they can achieve. To address the gap between risk and reward in the survey, new partnerships require that contracts spell out the opportunity for reward after improvement projects prove successful. To achieve this, clinical information is linked to an accounting model that calculates the exact savings associated with the specific improvements under contract. Reports on savings support the physician by providing motivation to sustain change after clarifying what percentage of an available bonus has been achieved. If the physicians question the data they should be able to interact with the report by clicking on an icon that moves the user to the next level of detail. For example, they may want to see the percentage of patients on the protocol or a comparison of their data with peers. Once physicians see the economics behind participation in an improvement protocol, they will support accelerated change.

On the clinical side, CIMCO reports should meet physicians' need for summary data that documents the success of efforts to improve outcomes. Once CIMCO has established credibility in the organization, it should have this level of dynamic reporting in place. When CIMCO can calculate the real dollar savings generated from successful implementation of clinical improvement projects as well as showing better clinical outcomes, physicians will treat specific education with enthusiasm. Physicians learn that techniques to cooperate in the specific delivery of care are necessary to achieve business strategies.

CIMCO's success is defined by its ability to gather, analyze, and report the data needed to align incentives fairly with what physicians say they want. CIMCO must draw on a portion of revenue for its operating expenses and then operate as a revenue center if the partnership is to sustain its operation. To ensure ongoing success, CIMCO must perform regular internal financial forecasts and audits, the results of which regularly communicate financial viability to the top executive leadership of the partnership.

## Closing the Gap Between Primary Care and Specialists

CIMCO can help foster collaboration between specialty and primary care physicians through its reports and educational focus. A true cooperative effort requires that both groups believe fairness is being achieved through clinical and fiscal accountability. Funds that are generated and used for reward will be the subject of conflict without cooperation from both sides on every project. What is most important is for both groups to understand and have a fair stake in revenue sharing. The legal contracts that manage the risk reward aspect of new relationships with physicians determine the rules. Defining fairness from a legal perspective varies state by state. Certificate of need, corporate practice of medicine, and other state legislation on physician ownership of hospitals will direct the options. New partnerships should also be careful to avoid violating Medicare regulations, including fraud and abuse, federal antitrust, Stark legislation, or Internal Revenue Service (IRS) regulations on inurement. As new revenue-sharing partnerships are tested in the courts there will be clearer guidance on how to structure these agreements.

The financial benefit of cooperation provides a powerful tool to unite a wide variety of providers across the partnership; however, each organization should stay within the agreed-upon constraints. Partnerships should obtain legal advice before instituting revenue-sharing plans. As long as the accounting for reward is accurately calculated by CIMCO and clinical data are accurate and clear, the legal risks can be managed.

### Supporting Behavioral Change

To build positive change, CIMCO must organize and direct the activities of providers who have never been in a large and complex partnership before. CIMCO must resolve old conflicts that exist because of poor communication, turf wars, and outdated assumptions. A major task of CIMCO will be using dialogue for both communication and education. CIMCO personnel will not only teach, but will also keep the office informed about where redesign and clinical improvement are needed. CIMCO supports new behavior by facilitating access to focused data, by analyzing it, and then reporting it to the physicians and managers. The office aggressively informs providers participating in CPI research efforts when a method of improving care has been proven to succeed. Individual providers then decide their level of involvement in each project. Specific education, facilitated meetings, and formal peer discussions are needed to support the CIMCO strategy every step of the way.

Collecting, organizing, purging, and analyzing data involves new data management discipline and requires focused support and commitment by management to the office's success. Organizations are always resistant to data collection and analysis. The strategies of the past information era are inadequate to achieve the level of coordination necessary for CIMCO. The issue of coordination and accountability must be formally addressed within a more interactive, yet safe environment via manuals, new job descriptions, task assignments, and timelines.

Once specific projects are under way, facts regarding the results of return on investment (ROI) projections are evaluated here. However, the actual reward function is not within CIMCO's purview. CIMCO guides physician behavior by reporting the achievement of projections approved by the steering committee. The system executives and the board members remain responsible for managing the contracts that spell out reward. If the partnership is to maintain accelerated change and credibility, CIMCO's work must receive high priority from this executive group. Supporting the expectations that are managed by CIMCO is the key to visible fairness and new physician behavior.

Keep in mind the office's sole responsibility is to carry out the complex tasks, previously discussed, to bring about accelerated improvement. Maintaining a clear and narrow focus is required if new physician behavior is to be achieved and sustained. This chapter has emphasized the need for structure to organize clinical change. The next chapter explains the method to redesign clinical care as a formal discipline using disease state management.

# 10

# Implementing a Project
# to Manage a Disease State

The previous chapter described the organizational infrastructure
needed to coordinate the use of data. This chapter will further
explore the work of the clinical information management and communication office (CIMCO) by detailing a practical method for
conducting a typical project to manage a disease state.

To understand the best use of CIMCO, search for a process for
disease state management in a specific, well-researched clinical area.
Asthma fits these criteria. CIMCO would begin with a feasibility
analysis (see Chapter Five for a full description). The first goal of
CIMCO would be to determine whether asthma is a good initial
project for disease state management, and it clearly is. For example,
asthma affects more than 12 million Americans, and costs of care
exceed $6 billion per year. Asthma is associated with the loss of nor-
mal social activity and work productivity.

This pulmonary disease is one of the areas that has already been
approached by the Institute for Healthcare Improvement and a
number of major health care systems such as Jewish Hospitals, Mayo
Clinic, Lovelace Health System, the University of Pennsylvania,
Health Partners, Allina, and others. All of these integrated systems
used some technique for feasibility assessment and clinical process
improvement similar to those described in Chapter Five. When this
much experience with a single disease begins to reach the literature,
the feasibility of a project is usually high.

The care for asthma is also a good choice for CIMCO because the care includes a wide variety of providers with varying expertise and diverse backgrounds based out of multiple locations. These multiple locations include the doctor's office, home health care, outpatient treatment centers, ER, ICU, and the hospital floor. Coordinating the information collection, clinical decision support, and financial analysis across all of these locations will force CIMCO to build a comprehensive data network that can be used to support other projects. Eventually CIMCO will track successful home health care, self-care, physician office care, and inpatient care. This allows a new approach to emerge across the continuum of care.

The best approach to outpatient and inpatient management of asthma has been measured, and national benchmarks exist. CIMCO staff reviews the literature on disease state management for best practices and benchmarks. On the Internet, one can also visit a variety of sites to search the asthma publications. They include www.nlm.nih.gov/databases/freemedl.html, which is a site created by the U.S. National Library of Medicine. It includes links to Grateful Med, PubMed, and Lonesome Docs. Www.ginasthma.com is a project conducted in collaboration with the National Heart, Lung, and Blood Institute, National Institute of Health, and the World Health Organization. Www.niaid.nih.gov is a site by the National Institute of Allergy and Infectious Diseases, hosted by the National Institute of Health, just to name a few.

CIMCO integrates the key facts from the literature and creates materials and reports to use for physician education later. CIMCO organizes the physicians to develop a process to improve asthma, including inpatient and outpatient management plans, ER protocols, self-care protocols, home health care instruction, and community outreach.

Next, CIMCO organizes a discussion involving all those professionals who interact to manage the disease. Key issues will include patient selection criteria for treatment, therapy selection, therapy duration, appropriate use of home health care, education, and a health status evaluation. Creating a care map or flow chart will help to clarify the feasibility of implementing the new process steps and capturing the needed data. Someone should facilitate the discussion to help the group to decide on first steps.

Assuming CIMCO and the professionals involved believe the project is initially feasible, they should construct a statement to support a simple hypothesis. For example, "If we provide education to the high-risk patient and place the patient and family on a home management protocol, it will decrease ER visits. If successful, we will prevent suffering of the patient and create savings."

### Projecting the Budget

It is essential to establish the CPI organizational plan and project a financial budget that could support the project for the first operating year. Before collecting any data, CIMCO should perform a profit-and-loss analysis and a ROI calculation. The CPI plan should identify available resources and estimate the cost of design, development, and full implementation (including the initial data collection and analysis). This profit-and-loss statement should include a financial projection of savings that can be reviewed at a later date to evaluate the project's success at financial forecasting.

For example, a small integrated delivery system in Texas with a 350–bed hospital and about 1,500 patients with asthma in their ER annually reviewed their data and made the following projections. They estimated that about two-thirds (or 1000) of visits were pediatric. Most of the collectible fees in this community are reimbursed under discounted fee-for-service contracts. The total ER charges per visit were just under $700. By reviewing the literature, they made some assumptions. W. L. McNabb used an intervention with children and families that cost $180 per child and reduced the number of ER visits per child from 7.4 to 1.9. This improvement reduced visits to 25.6 percent of the original volume (McNabb and others, 1986, pp. 103–107). If the Texas hospital could reproduce this success with the 135 high-risk children in their pediatric case load, they could drop the ER visits to approximately 250 and prevent about 750 visits.

Because the hospital was already tracking unit-based variable costs from the ER separated out by diagnosis-related group (DRG) and current procedural terminology (CPT) code, they could calculate their real cost. They subtracted their collections on the ER services delivered from their real costs to determine whether they currently profited or lost money providing care to this population. It turned out that their overall collections on asthma patients seen in the ER were only 50 percent. By comparing real costs to collections it was clear that the hospital lost about $50 on average per visit.

The cost of the educational intervention to prevent the targeted ER visits was estimated to be $180 per patient. With 135 patients the total cost came to $24,300. If they prevented 750 ER visits through education, they would save the hospital $37,500 in direct reductions of variable costs. These variable costs were the real costs of care not being covered by collections. Because of increasing ER volume as a result of the system's successful growth in market share, the ER physicians were not likely to lose any actual revenue, so physician complaints were unlikely. To see patients in the office rather than in the ER was another positive benefit for the practice, since they operated under a fee-for-service plan. This additional revenue also had to be tracked and reported.

The rough estimate of ROI for the hospital was savings of $37,500 minus $24,300 for educational intervention for a total savings of $13,200. This is a 64.8 percent return on the $24,300 investment. Although the savings were relatively small, the ROI percentage was impressive enough to at least consider the project. The team knew there would be other probable costs such as meetings and data management. As they listed other costs, they calculated the average ER cost if the remaining 250 asthma admits were more severely ill on average than current asthma patients. It wasn't long before the $13,200 potential savings had been lost.

The feasibility projection also included an estimate of what the insurance companies would save by not having to pay for the insured patients' ER visits. If 750 visits were eliminated, it would have saved the avoided ER charges that would normally go to the insurance company. They multiplied the number of avoided ER charges by the percentage of patients covered by insurance. About 57 percent of patients actually had insurance. This amount was multiplied by the percentage of reimbursement paid by the carrier, about 75 percent. This created a total savings of $224,437 for the insurance company, even though they did not support the funding or the improvement effort. The insurer added no value to the project, yet they would receive the bonus.

The team recognized that some cost shifting would occur with more office visits being traded for less ER visits. Any shift in self-medication would also add cost. As they continued their feasibility analysis, they considered the losses the hospital would experience from prevented hospital admits under fee for service. The third party clearly benefited more from these savings than the original estimate. The reward for the third party was many times the cost of the improved disease management. However, the hospital part of the partnership would actually lose money in fee for service to carry out the DSM project because they would not share in these savings.

### Finding Motivation to Change Payers

With a shared risk contract, the amount calculated as a benefit to the third party is added to the profit side of the profit-and-loss sheet. The cost of the improvement subtracted from this amount gives the return on investment. Even if the educational interventions were to cost twice the budgeted amount, as long as the partnership kept the savings it would be inspiring rather than unfair. Subtracting the revenue from new office visits would cause the project to fall slightly short of the original budget. Even in the previous example, this calculation would still give a ROI of well over $100,000 on the original $24,300 spent to conduct the intervention.

This analysis proves just how broken the current health care system is. The delivery system in Texas will find it hard to implement this project because it requires an economic sacrifice on the part of the providers. Until the new practice of medicine removes the financial risk from trying to improve the community's health, real improvement will be understandably slow.

*Sharing Risk as a Strategy*

The Texas facility is implementing a strategy that forces the hospital to create an artificial reward for the physician partners. Their goal is to build a culture of physicians that believe in prevention by stimulating successful disease state management with reward and by tracking the debt that is accrued. Next they must promote their own insurance product or partner with an insurance company until they are large enough to benefit from the savings they create in this product. Once the savings are enough to outweigh the losses that they are suffering by providing DSM under traditional insurance contracts, their strategy for success will be complete. This strategy may sound difficult, but for physician–hospital partnerships that have 50 percent of their patients covered by Medicare or Medicaid, the transition is getting easier. Many feel that the government is likely to freeze its health care spending and encourage insurance companies and hospital systems to compete for full-risk contracts. If these government populations move to coverage that is capitated via a fixed budget HMO model, the volume of patients available for coverage under an at-risk partnership product is more than enough to succeed. The problem will be the size of the fixed payment. If it falls well below the current insurance rates, the savings disappear. The key for this Texas-based integrated delivery system is to increase the market share of their own insurance product quickly before the budgeted revenues drop too low.

If a partnership has at least 30 percent of their patients in capitated contracts such as Medicaid and Medicare HMOs, they can implement this model without being inhibited by economics. The challenge for these partnerships is implementing good projects for disease state management, cost accounting, and motivating physician involvement.

If the profit-and-loss analysis for a DSM project can include the third party savings, the project will most likely be a financial success. The asthma project used as an example would be highly profitable for the system and the community if the $224,437 could be kept locally rather than benefiting the third party. A retrospective analysis or review of existing baselines before a project is launched can project savings from improvement and also demonstrate that the improvement effort will not increase the morbidity of patients included in the study. The retrospective analysis provides the partnership with an assessment of the barriers that will be encountered during the prospective phase of the CPI project. After the first phase of implementation, the resources needed to make the project successful and the baseline for clinical and financial comparisons can be more accurately defined.

CIMCO constructs the prospective research design with clinical information and the help of the physicians who will provide the care. Implementation will be conducted in several practices by using a sequence developed by a CPI team. Like the educational intervention in the example, the project itself must start simply and then expand to include areas such as treatment choice in the ER, the office of the PCPs, an allergy or asthma center, and the hospital. CIMCO will be involved in organizing and tracking the processes being implemented. This implementation tracking function should be displayed in a graphic form on a report as a percentage of possible steps taken or of total patients participating.

Reports should show the physicians what percentage of their goals they are currently achieving in parallel with the percentage of the eligible bonus they have been receiving. As clinical care changes, CIMCO reviews these reports to look for any shifting of costs across the continuum of care that are present in the past data. One challenge is learning to see how the economic losses in one part of the partnership creates success in another part of the system.

### Goals for Asthma Disease State Management

A group of physicians in New Mexico who accomplished a simple project to improve their approach to asthma developed a list of goals. They said they would expand their improvement efforts sequentially by adding one goal as soon as the previous goal had been accomplished. The goals to be implemented were

- Improving the health of the individual through self-participation in healthy behaviors.

- Improving the patient compliance with self-treatment and awareness of the circumstances that represent a need to intervene in problem areas.

- Using visual displays to give feedback to patients about performance of key processes of care (for example, peak flow values).

- Improving patient-provider communication across the continuum of care, including counseling and education.

- Improving the provider's knowledge of the patient's lifestyle and status without increasing the provider's workload by successfully assisting the patient and patient's family with data gathering, interpretation, and compliance.

- Identifying areas of patient care not in compliance with national practice guidelines. (This step can be accomplished through computerized decision support with data from electronic medical records and a health risk assessment, but it could also be done on paper.)

- Allowing individual providers confidentially to compare themselves to all other providers and supplying education to raise performance where appropriate. (This area overlaps with quality assurance but must be handled as education, not as an issue for individual credentialing.)

- Authorizing the system to rate the overall health status of this population of patients, practice by practice, as compared to benchmarks.

These complex goals are more likely to be achieved if they are added separately as each requires their own support.

CIMCO could help implement and manage each of these DSM goals eventually, but it will do so by adding one step at a time. By succeeding at the implementation of an easy earlier step, like documenting the depth of participation in education, CIMCO can more easily add additional goals. For example, the next step might be to do a risk screening on all of the at-risk patients in each of the practices. Once that DSM project is mature the national practice guidelines can be added, but that level of complexity is never a first step.

### Launching the Disease State Management Project

All communication methods—newsletters, telephone, and the Internet—can be used to coordinate care for patients across the multiple encounters, providers, and settings that define care for a single disease. Ideally, this communication is organized with the development of national treatment guidelines that have been adapted for local use. The steps needed to launch the DSM program are as follows:

- CIMCO staff presents the program to the care providers and identifies the project champions.

- CIMCO staff evaluates local resources available for the program and for the program steering committee.

- A team composed of the key physicians, visiting nurses, hospital personnel, pharmacists, respiratory therapists, pharmaceutical representatives, and school nurses agrees on simple guidelines taken from the literature.

- A multidisciplinary working team of the people that will adapt and develop the program is formed. They usually function as a subset of the steering committee.

- The working team reviews the literature to determine what questions are important. They generate specific clinical and financial questions for the DSM after learning how to use the Internet to obtain summaries of clinical articles. They then evaluate the quality of the literature.

- The team creates a financial model to reward providers based upon compliance with the DSM program. Reward is based on compliance, not outcomes. This addresses the problem of severity adjustment because physicians should not be penalized if their patient has a bad outcome even though they did the right thing.

- Questionnaires are administered to providers to assess current treatment practices, knowledge of national recommendations, and their willingness to adopt a distributed-care model.

- The team develops a baseline of current health care delivery and resource utilization to show improvement.

- Existing populations are defined and evaluated with administrative data, pharmacy billing data, and hospital data. Patients with an asthmatic history or an unsure designation receive a survey administered as a self-reported questionnaire. The results stratify the patient into one of four classes of asthma: mild, mild persistent, moderate persistent, and severe persistent. A fifth class is unknown severity. The PCP then receives a list of their patients with a tentative severity group designation and the results of their responses.

- The practice groups the patients by severity to target the planned interventions and decide who to target first.

- Asthmatics are contacted depending on the priority that is established. One possible schedule is shown in Figure 10.1.

**Figure 10.1. Schedule for Patient Follow-Up in Asthma DSM.**

| Severity | Home Visit | Phone Visit | See Provider | Group Education |
|---|---|---|---|---|
| Mild | | • q 6 mo | • X1 and PRN | • q 1 yr |
| Mild persistent | | • q 3 mo | • XI and q 6 mo | • q 6 mo |
| Moderate persistent | • q 3 mo | •q 1 mo | • q 3 mo? | • q 3 mo |
| Severe persistent | • q 1–3 mo | • q mo when not visited | • q 2 mo? | • q 2 mo |
| Unsure | | • to assess severity | • X1 and others based on severity | • |

*Key:* q = every time; X = times.
*Source:* Courtesy of Jim Frankfurt, M.D., FCCP

- The team develops specific educational interventions and protocols for patients based on whether the patient is compliant with care guidelines. The first educational interventions should be simple, such as relevant reading materials, personalized phone calls, and computerized feedback.

- Education is provided in workshops and through home health educators. The targets are the high-risk patients, the family, and other support groups that have been identified. The team uses handouts and a variety of data collection tools. A self-coded data sheet is developed by CIMCO staff to track results. It is important to keep the first pass simple (as illustrated in Figure 10.2). This one-page sheet is intentionally lacking in any real detail.

- Program rollout timelines are developed for each office or site where the program can be piloted.

- Practice guidelines, clinical pathways, algorithms, and forms are refined. Team consensus is important to this process, especially when the guidelines are generated in the face of insufficient evidence from the literature. If evidence cannot be found in the literature, then pathophysiological rationale, clinical judgment, and local utilization data have to play a role.

- The program is rolled out to pilot offices or sites.

- Data is collected for a defined number of patients.

- Data is analyzed and reports are prepared. Figures 10.3 and 10.4 are examples of sample reports.

- The steering committee or CIMCO reviews the pilot project's success as described in the reports.

- The decision to implement a broad rollout of DSM according to a timeline is considered.

**Figure 10.2. Self-Coded Data Sheet.**

## Inpatient Information

Patient Name: _____

Hospital [ ][ ]     173 = Hospital A
                    221 = Hospital B
                    765 = Hospital C

Patient Birth date #: [ ][ ] M M [ ][ ] D D [ ][ ] Y Y

Admit Date: [ ][ ] [ ][ ] [ ][ ]

Discharge Date: [ ][ ] [ ][ ] [ ][ ]

Medical Record #: [ ][ ][ ][ ][ ][ ]

Pt. Account #: [ ][ ][ ][ ][ ][ ]

Male [ ]    Female [ ]

## Outpatient Information

Clinic Visit Date: [ ][ ] [ ][ ] [ ][ ]

Date of Education: [ ][ ] [ ][ ] [ ][ ]

CPT Code [ ][ ][ ]

ICD-9 Code for Primary Surgical Procedure: [ ][ ][ ]

Socioeconomic Status [ ]     1 = Low Income
                             2 = Med/High Income
                             3 = Unavailable
                             4 = Unknown

Asthma Risk: [ ]     1 = Low
                     2 = High
                     3 = Unavailable
                     4 = Unknown

Case Class: [ ]     1 = Elective
                    2 = Urgent
                    3 = Emergent
                    7 = Unavailable
                    9 = Unknown

**Figure 10.2. Self-Coded Data Sheet, Cont'd.**

| | Date | | | Military Time |
|---|---|---|---|---|
| Date and time patient entered ER: | | | | : |
| Date and time patient discharged from ER: | | | | : |
| Date and time patient entered holding: | | | | : |
| Date and time patient discharged from holding: | | | | : |
| | M M | D D | Y Y | H H M M |

## Treatment Information

| | | |
|---|---|---|
| High Risk Self Care Protocol Given: | ☐ | 1 = Yes<br>2 = No<br>7 = Unavailable<br>9 = Unknown |
| Child Care Protocol Given: | ☐ | 1 = Yes<br>2 = No<br>7 = Unavailable<br>9 = Unknown |
| Asthma Treatment Protocol Followed: | ☐ | 1 = Yes<br>2 = No<br>7 = Unavailable<br>9 = Unknown |
| Home Care Treatment Given: | ☐ | 1 = Yes<br>2 = No<br>7 = Unavailable<br>9 = Unknown |

## Figure 10.3. Sample SAGE™ Summary DSM Report.

---

### Success at a Glance Evidence
#### Confidential Detail Report of DSM: Asthma Feb. '98

For: Individual Physician Code 273633
Re: Personal Data

---

Average number of asthmatics followed = 55.
Average percentage of practice = 5%. Participant since 6/1/97.

| Outcome | # Patients | Benchmark Result | Group PAQ Result | Your Result | p > .05 PAQ | P >.05 Bench |
|---|---|---|---|---|---|---|
| % w/ Management plans | 50 | 100 | 85 | 96 | + | |
| % Using peak flow | 30 | 100 | 60 | 75 | + | − |
| % on Anti-inflammatory meds | 45 | 100 | 75 | 90 | + | |
| % on Theophyllines | 10 | 10 | 50 | 20 | − | + |
| % ED visits | 50 | 0 | 15 | 5 | − | |
| % Hosp admissions | 50 | 0 | 10 | 2.5 | | |
| % in control | 50 | 100 | 87 | 95 | | |
| % Education | 50 | 100 | 80 | 92 | + | |
| Cost (PMPM) | 50 | 30 | 42 | 28 | − | |

Statistics: + indicates statistically greater
− indicates statistically less than comparison group

### Asthma DSM Measurements Q2/97. Comparative Results

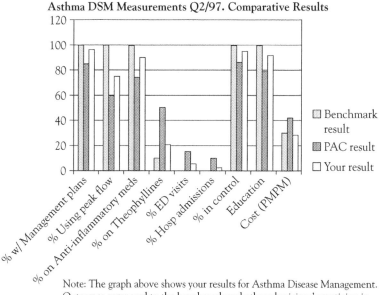

Note: The graph above shows your results for Asthma Disease Management.
Outcomes compared to the benchmark and other physicians' practicing in
PAQs. Statistical comparisons are located in the table above.

The top table shows the breakdown of an individual physician's asthma DSM
outcomes. All the outcomes are reported as a percentage of total patients who got
the intervention. This is then compared to the benchmark and other physicians
in the group. The total number of patients and statistical significance are also
totaled. The bar graph shows comparisons of benchmark, group result, and the
individual result side by side for each outcome.

## Figure 10.4. Sample SAGE™ of a Detailed DSM Report.

---

**Success at a Glance Evidence**
*Confidential Detail Report of DSM: Asthma Feb. '98*

For: Individual Physician Code 273633
Re: Personal Data

---

| Percentage on | | |
|---|---|---|
| **Month** | **Anti-Inflammatory** | **P < .05** |
| 3/97 | 43 | – |
| 4/97 | 47 | – |
| 5/97 | 51 | – |
| 6/97 | 49 | – |
| 7/97 | 54 | – |
| 8/97 | 60 | – |
| 9/97 | 63 | – |
| 10/97 | 60 | – |
| 11/97 | 72 | |
| 12/97 | 71 | – |
| 1/98 | 87 | |
| 2/98 | 90 | |

Average number of asthmatics
followed = 55
Average percentage of practice = 5%
Participant since 6/1/97
Date of this report: 6/12/98

• This is a measure of the percentage
of all asthmatics on anti-inflammatory
meds.

• Statistics:
+ indicates statistically greater
– indicates statistically less than
benchmark value (p<.05)

**Anti-Inflammatory Use**

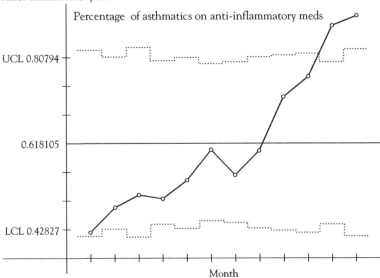

This report is a more detailed look at one outcome measure, percentage anti-inflammatory medications given to the patient population over one year. The SPC chart shows the process improvement to be significantly better as a trend.

**Adding Additional Data**

Additional data for a more detailed follow-up are added to the collection tool only if they are needed to document success as the roll-out expands. Additional data could include

- A more detailed health risk assessment

- Disease-specific health risk and compliance assessment

- Data collection of disease-specific variables (peak flow, medication, and so forth)

- Data display of trends

Some approaches that use technology include

- Computerized asthma practice guidelines for the patient and the provider

- Real-time decision support (alerts and reminders)

- Knowledge-authoring tools to code practice guidelines

- Databases regarding the use of educational material for patient and provider that outlines disease care and compliance

- Databases outlining what patient information was given and a log of what interventions were used

- Vocabulary mapping between the system's IS department and new terminology used in the project to support the exchange of patient data between the health compliance records and the system's clinical records

Human effort and paper processing can replace the high-technology approach. The manual project is just as viable; it simply takes more time and effort to maintain speed and accuracy. CIMCO should not wait for full electronic support to begin, but should anticipate what support will be needed. All data collection tools should also be compatible with future strategic IS plans.

### Sustaining the Gains of the Improvement Strategy

As the improvement is implemented, a detailed, ongoing quarterly review and analysis of data and reporting—whether it is electronic or paper—are needed to focus on current measures of clinical information and outcomes, data support capabilities, and implementation and monitoring abilities for improving quality. Bimonthly meetings on process improvement should be held with physicians, clinicians, managers, and other staff who are involved in launching the initial projects and whose support will be essential to the ongoing implementation of the improvement. In addition, the steering committee should receive a quarterly report regarding the recommended changes to the implemented program. A timeline should be created to track project implementation. A check-off list of milestones can easily be developed to assist process change and track the effectiveness of implementation for each study.

As a final step in the reporting process, the unit-based cost data are applied to results, and the return on investment or economic losses are tracked. Accurate and in-depth financial projections are critical elements in the opening phases of the project. Management will be comfortable rewarding providers, even though there is a delay in the return on investment, as long as they can see how long before the project earns a ROI. One of the most important steps in this process is disseminating the results in clear reports. Figure 10.5 is an example of this type of clear financial report.

### Priorities

During the first year of CIMCO operation, target populations are identified based on key indicators such as volume of patients with a specific disease, the cost of their care, and the likelihood that a

**Figure 10.5. Sample of a Summary Report for the Hospital Partner.**

| Success at a Glance Evidence |
| :---: |
| *Confidential Summary Report of DSM Results July '98* |
| For: Partnership Steering Committee |
| Re: Hospital Partner Code: 273633 |

| DSM Achievement: | | | |
| --- | --- | --- | --- |
| | DSM Goals | 48% | ☆ |
| | Financial Goals | 53% | |
| | Cost Savings | $456,265 | |
| **Clinical Effectiveness:** | | | |
| | Incentive Bonus | $113,322 | ☆ |
| Percentage of Max Achievable | | 50% | |
| **Productivity:** | | | |
| | Number of Visits | 14,830 | |
| | Number of Procedures | 625 | |
| **Satisfaction:** | | | |
| | Patient Satisfaction | 95% | |
| | Perception of Access | 98% | |
| **Income Trend:** | | | |
| Current trend has improved to a statistically significant degree. Month to month variation remains high and overall percentage of max achievable bonus remains well below benchmark | | | |

☆ = significant trend exists in component of this group.

This report shows the summaries of the key indicators that were important to the partnership steering committee in looking at all hospital-based DSM projects. The percentage of goals achieved as well as financial goals are listed together with total dollars saved under Clinical Effectiveness. The incentives achieved correlate with the DSM goals achieved. Total visits and procedures are listed under Productivity. Patient Satisfaction and Perception of Access are high, but the Income Trend, even though improving at a statistically significant rate, is far from its full potential.

fixed payment for the population's care can be achieved. Because Medicaid and Medicare are turning to fixed budgets for reimbursement state by state, this category of patients may warrant special consideration in most areas.

The following list of diagnoses represents 80 percent of the cost and volume of disease treatment in integrated health care delivery systems.

Different regions will have specific opportunities not listed here, and the list of successful improvement is growing rapidly (Gutman, 1999). Because disease state management (DSM) has been slow to move into the outpatient setting, many of the major diagnoses reviewed in the literature are those requiring inpatient care. These specialty projects provide the focus for the early process improvements that create hospital-based savings. It doesn't matter what type of project the partnership starts with, as long as they use the early DSM developmental projects as a springboard to go beyond hospital care to the full continuum.

**Exhibit 10.1.  Targets for Disease State Management.**

Systemwide Disease Management Projects
Cover 80% of Health System Cost and Patient Volume

| | | |
|---|---|---|
| Allergic rhinitis | CABG | Hypertension |
| Alzheimer's | Chest pain | Joint injury |
| Antibiotic management | Colon-related cancer | Low back pain |
| Anticoagulation | Congestive heart failure | Osteoporosis |
| Anxiety | Decubitus ulcers | Otitis media |
| Aspiration pneumonia | Deep vein thrombosis | Pregnancy management |
| Asthma | Dementia | Prostate cancer |
| Arthritis | Depression | Schizophrenia |
| Attention deficit disorder | Diabetes | Stroke |
| Birth management | Epilepsy | Substance abuse |
| Breast cancer | Hyperlipidemia | Total hip replacement |

### Learning from Evaluation

The CIMCO or equivalent operational division over DSM is responsible to formalize feedback and manage communication to ensure learning.

Evaluation of the success of the new partnerships as well as individual project performance and reward requires measurement. Communication and information exchange must be accomplished at logical intervals over time to facilitate learning and change. Although annual reports are helpful for planning and tracking trends, quarterly and even monthly reports of physicians' success, demonstrating significant trends, are a necessity to sustain enthusiasm and behavioral change. The principles of CPI measurement (as described in Chapter Five) guide the evaluation and documentation of the DSM process. By standardizing the reporting process and using consistent graphic methods to illustrate the DSM process and achievements, physicians will understand what leads to organizational and team-wide cooperation. Detailing the project's progress and success will propel the change process.

Accountability for completing tasks on a schedule needs to be managed in a nonpunitive way. The steps necessary to achieve success on the job can be established and improved by following a variety of methods. If the above steps are taken, and the evaluation shows what support is needed, progress is achieved as support is added. CIMCO's job is to fix problems of implementation to ensure the success of disease state management. The data collection is directed toward known success factors, and these are defined as measurable steps needed to make continual progress.

Inertia and delay in DSM projects indicate problems. They cannot be ignored because they point to an error in direction or to failed support. CIMCO responds to these warning signs through a systematic redesign effort. Comparing delays to projections of savings will show the real cost of delay in dollars lost month by month.

Several critical internal categories of measurement are used to prove the real success of disease state management. The cost of work conducted, cost of care provided, and contracts relating to revenue (fee for service versus capitation) must be considered. The cost of completing the project is calculated as a proportion of the total real costs. This is then compared to projections as an internal check on the economic effectiveness of the DSM project. The process steps that are successfully changed can also be measured as a percentage of the total number of steps that could have been changed. This gives the CIMCO steering committee an idea of the effectiveness of the CPI or DSM team. The number of errors in care can also become a specific target for improvement by tracking the delays or omissions in care steps and relating them to the important clinical outcomes. Satisfaction, cost, and clinical outcomes are also measured and linked through cause-and-effect relationships.

A formal evaluation of cross-disciplinary input and the provider response to new information can be tracked as a measure of system integration. Assessments of the impact of a DSM project on other services can be specific or subjective. The attitude and participation of medical staff can be assessed individually, by department, or systemwide.

Data collection, the completed analysis, and the percentage of protocol steps followed all measure whether success will be accomplished according to the timeline. CIMCO also tracks the percentage of the projected outcome achieved and the percentage of the results sustained over time. In addition, the projected budget is compared to the actual cost, and savings are compared to the amount allocated for implementation to see whether the expected savings have been created. The success or failure of a DSM project is based on clinical and financial facts that change in response to new behavior. CIMCO's evaluation of the success of disease state management provides a learning opportunity for the physicians, and physicians' feedback leads to new DSM strategies and learning opportunities for CIMCO.

### Learning About Each Other

After a successful infrastructure is in place and DSM projects are expected to succeed, the partnership can support education that accelerates new physician and management behavior. This requires changing old expectations toward the constant improvement described here. Failing to help physicians accept change represents the greatest stumbling block to the successful integration of health care systems. Individuals in the new partnerships can use self-education, which requires specific projects, clear data, trust, and a commitment to open two-way communication. Physicians willing to risk change must learn of its benefits. This step requires a DSM structure and information that make the opportunity to experiment safe. The freedom to experiment reassures physicians as they build the new interdependent practice of medicine (described as high performance in Chapter Six). Physicians need an operational plan and cooperation-based management to carry out these high-performance steps. Practices that are accountable for quality (PAQs) need CIMCO to broaden the power of continuous learning. PAQs are the clinical business units that implement the DSM and CPI strategies of CIMCO throughout the system and are a critical area to explore.

In this chapter, a detailed approach to managing the disease state has been described. This method can accelerate clinical improvements through organizing information and fostering motivation. The doctor's office presents the biggest challenge but is also the most important business unit influenced by this approach. The next chapter explores how a PAQ implements best office practice with the appropriate reward mechanism in place. To thrive and still do what is right, PAQs are organizing to lead the new health care partnerships. With the right approach and support, PAQs can learn to master the skills needed to lead the transformation to the new practice of medicine.

# 11

# Practices Accountable for Quality

The previous chapter detailed how information and operational support can be applied to disease state management to greatly enhance clinical work within the new health care partnerships. In this chapter, we move to the physicians' office and describe the operational structure needed to help physicians and their employees succeed in changing the direct delivery of outpatient care. These physician practices will be referred to as practices accountable for quality, or PAQs.

In all of the successful new health care partnerships that Medical Resource Management has helped redesign, the pressure of organizing accountable working groups of physicians has been an ever-present challenge. These practices are committed to using knowledge to achieve a new level of performance and reward. Changing physician behavior is difficult. First, the new practice must overcome the physicians' fear of using data to measure success. Data can document success, but it can also prove embarrassing, or jeopardize the ability of physicians to qualify for payer contracts. Therefore PAQs must agree to uniform operating structures and incentive systems and, most important, they must foster an environment of trust.

Using all six dimensions of physician leadership, new health care partnerships should be able to find mutual support and the structure to transform their medical practice. A small, accountable business unit is necessary to implement the new knowledge. Using the PAQ structure, it is also possible to integrate new frontline clinical information into a broad partnership. Unfortunately, most partnerships have not formally developed PAQs.

Physicians can get organized, find commitment, and sustain motivation by focusing on the cooperative strength of a small group. All of the separate PAQs can be organized by using information and incentives in a functional system.

Integrated systems began purchasing practices to create large physician-hospital partnerships in the 1990s. Through this process, it became apparent that building trust within these large groups of physicians was an overwhelming challenge (Lumsdom, 1996, p. 26). The massive size and attendant lack of accountability of these efforts has weakened many emerging integrated systems. PAQs offer a solution. For instance, whereas a group of 100 physicians of various specialties often cannot agree on policies, twenty small groups of five physicians are able to find agreement. Bound by the integrated approach to data (Chapter Three) and fair incentives (Chapter Four), these small groups become change agents for the new practice of medicine.

PAQs strive to accomplish the goals of efficiency in all areas of care and improved health of the patient. The hospital receives a reward for activities such as discharge planning because they help the PAQ create savings. Primary care physicians are rewarded for proper referrals to specialists that reduce unnecessary care. The specialists are rewarded for making efficient and cost-effective choices for the care they provide. The patient is rewarded by reduced premiums, and the community is rewarded by a healthier population. In some cases, the community benefits further from its economic investments in the future. When these concepts are directed by an economically defined operating unit of physicians (PAQ) willing to experiment, transformation becomes possible.

The PAQs must first define themselves, however. Physicians who trust each other must get organized to create a PAQ. The larger partnership is responsible for providing education to their physicians to organize them to form PAQs. Partnerships should use legal counsel and data support (such as CIMCO) to define visible fairness as it relates to these PAQs. In a large group of 300 physicians, there could be as many as 60 fundamental work units or PAQs, each employing their own staff. The partnership's challenge is one of coordinating these PAQs within the overall strategy for change. The practice is responsible for managing care and ensuring that the aligned incentives for its providers are fairly distributed. By tracking patient satisfaction and documenting overall improvement achieved by the PAQ, the partnership removes the fear of being unfairly accused of wrongdoing when economic pressures force system changes.

Resistance and anger were common reactions from physicians who were told they could be better providers through large, impersonal system-quality departments. This negative approach to physicians is replaced by a new focus on uniform support and cooperation. True integration of the partnership will occur only if coordinated support of small group practices is in place.

## The PAQ Guiding Principles

The guiding principles of the PAQ concept can be viewed as the specific areas that lend themselves to focused education. These key areas that can be measured, reported, improved, and rewarded are

- Aligning incentives for reimbursement

- Providing optimal support services

- Involving patients in care

- Achieving optimal utilization of resources

- Providing data support for clinical decision making

- Providing best patient care

- Evaluating clinical improvements

All of the key dimensions of physician leadership are used by the PAQ. But the seven work categories listed above define specific operational areas that the PAQ can improve. Proper redesign of these operations ensures that the PAQ will be both accountable to and successful for the partnership. Although the tools used to achieve success in these areas of work are relatively simple and represent widely accepted principles in theory, their implementation is always a challenge. The real work is in getting successful, well-educated decision makers to accept new knowledge (Argyris and Kaplan, 1994, p. 83).

Implementation of a PAQ overcomes resistance to change by placing successful, small-group cooperation first and foremost. PAQ physicians focus on unit-based cost accounting, clinical care tracking, and improvement, resulting in a commitment to embrace change. PAQ principles can be learned, but the greater contribution is that the PAQ creates expectations that cannot be forced on physicians by a large organization. To succeed, the large system must define aligned incentives attached to the PAQ's reimbursement for the desired clinical result. The PAQ addresses its own resistance to change. The physicians experiment, generate data, drive analysis, and capture the potential for reward together as a practice. The partnership simply provides the needed support, as described in the previous chapters.

The methods described in this chapter can be employed to achieve success within any integrated system. The principles of the PAQ are universal: They apply to all levels of the patient care continuum. In the office setting, the practice maximizes what physicians can do and minimizes nonproductive physician activities. These principles ask the practice to maximize customer satisfaction and minimize overhead. The PAQ principles help the physicians maximize data-driven decisions and minimize subjective decisions. The PAQ proves that information creates the cornerstone for the success of the new partnerships.

The partnership must manage multiple PAQs if the CIMCO or information support office is to be functional. The PAQ's data are critical if the partnership is to cost account for all activities. Supported by CIMCO, the PAQ is able to collect specific process and outcomes data that would otherwise escape the partnership. The methods and structures described under the following headings are the work areas that operationalize the grassroots changes critical to the PAQ. This work, combined with partnership support, is critical for the new health care partnership.

### Aligning Incentives for Reimbursement

For the PAQ to succeed, physicians must overcome the barriers to the implementation of new practice strategies. It would be naive to assume that just measuring care would be enough to facilitate change, or that incentives will accomplish change single-handedly. Physicians must also learn about clinical improvement methods and high-performance team skills. They must also believe that these new skills are valid and useful. When these changes are implemented, physicians must be supported in their work. Most important, physicians must overcome their own defensive and negative feelings about change. To meet this last challenge, physicians must find a sense of meaning behind the new work. Physicians who see each other as partners are motivated to make change. Aligning incentives in these small, accountable PAQs gives physicians the motivation to change, so it is this first PAQ principle on which partnerships should concentrate.

The PAQ understands that every service has a cost. In its drive to maximize quality and efficiency, the PAQ uses cost accounting as a framework for all critical decisions that affect reimbursement. Each step of medical care—from answering the telephone to prescribing antibiotics—has an associated cost. These costs are either fixed or variable, direct or indirect. Therefore, by applying simple accounting principles such as break-even analysis and calculating the contribution margin (revenue minus variable expenses) for a clinical product line, it is possible for the practice to track the flow of money. The income will vary widely because of reimbursement from different types of managed care contracts in the same practice.

Achieving aligned incentives requires analyzing all of the contracts for variation in reimbursement. For example, if the payment mechanism is fee-for-service (FFS), expenses are subtracted from the revenue until a break-even point is reached, after which more care creates profit. Under the FFS model, more is better. Under capitation, the same high volume of care only makes a profit when triage, education, and even home care are added to the continuum so that patients can avoid expensive care. This allows the practice to see a larger number of covered lives while keeping the cost of total care under the original budget. Financial losses are seen when the financial analysis required to track success won't cover the variable costs of additional care. If costs reach the break-even point with the revenues, more care creates a loss without adding revenue. This attention to appropriate accounting and financial forecasting replaces the old thinking, "We should take this contract because we need the patients."

When PAQs partner together, they can contract as a single large group and have leverage with a major payer. For many physicians, this leverage is the greatest value of the partnership. Properly managed, the new partnerships ensure that the appropriate reimbursement opportunities can be achieved. However, to succeed under the opportunity of shared risk, the PAQs must be able to manage their own governance, fees, benefits, and business processes. Each PAQ must align their own incentives and overcome conflict. Because the PAQ remains small and functional, these physicians guide each other through the shift in thinking required to share risk.

The PAQ succeeds by providing incentives to its own physicians under shared-risk reimbursement even if all the physicians are specialists. However, specialists face a unique risk when they accept a cap on spending. Not only are the physicians responsible for medical management of the patients for whom they provide care, but they are also responsible for appropriate referrals by primary care physicians. Specialists' concern is that when they are capitated outside of primary care the primary care physicians (PCPs) may no longer manage routine problems within the specialist realm, even though this care used to be included in the upper end of primary care. To prevent this behavior, protocols defining transfer of care based on symptoms and the results of specific tests need to be developed. The other alternative is to plan on the specialist taking on this higher level primary care and the revenue estimated to cover this care. Specialists need to be reimbursed for providing care to this population or PCPs need to continue their original practice pattern. This problem, often called the *dumping syndrome*, only occurs when individual PAQs are not willing to cooperate with each other.

The cause is usually the issue of reimbursement. Under the new practice of medicine, PCPs and specialists define fair cooperative contracts and relationships. Cooperation must be maintained because of the financial shifting that occurs as care is delivered under new strategies. Formal meetings and education to explain data are needed to reinforce the commitment to visible fairness.

The specialists' PAQs work out the proper referral guidelines for their high-end care with the PCPs' PAQs. Not only does the pre-specialist care delivered by the PCPs need to be complete, but also the records need to be transferred as soon as the patients shift their care from one provider to another. Communication between the two groups improves the specialists' outcomes and expedites decision making. PAQs need to agree on the accounting and clinical process steps that should be tracked. If the physicians are grouped into PAQs, and each PAQ is succeeding, the cooperation within all the groups will improve.

### Providing Optimal Support Services

PAQs do not simply evolve out of the present system. They are created from a disciplined effort to develop new skills and new relationships. The implementation of support services such as CIMCO are critical, but support within the PAQ is also important. For instance, emergency departments have long used nurses to provide triage based on patient acuity. Adapting this successful ER support model can help PAQs to streamline their own practice by adding triage. Many PAQs also added after-hours telephone support, a service that has been used by many hospitals and health plans for years. If the practice takes a contract to be at-risk for the cost of care through a fixed budget, helping patients achieve appropriate access to medical services becomes an economic necessity. For example, keeping patients out of the ER and getting them to the right provider as soon as possible becomes a necessary improvement and a critical business strategy.

There are two conditions that influence how the triage personnel deal with patient appointments. The first relates to the previous history of compliance with a published appointment guidelines schedule. In this case, the receptionist may call the patient to come in. In the second instance, the patient may insist on an appointment to evaluate a health problem, and the patient initiates the call. In either case, a physician completes a short questionnaire after each patient encounter that allows the physician to record whether the appointment was necessary or unnecessary, or should have been triaged to another provider. For example, a practice in Massachusetts began using a pen-pad data-entry device to capture this type of data by touching the boxes on a screen with specially prepared simple bullets listed in a column. As each patient care encounter was concluded, the boxes in the hand-held electronic pad were checked so that the results could automatically be entered into a confidential database. Reviewed monthly, these data helped the practice confidentially track the success of its own evolving triage system.

Similar to the way insurance companies attempt to manage the level of medical care through preauthorization, the PAQ delineates its own care guidelines. These care guidelines are used by all levels of office staff to decide what level of medical care is needed for each patient. The PAQ's care guidelines direct the staff and physicians in scheduling, referral, follow-up, and most medical care. These utilization guidelines will determine the real medical needs of the population across a complex health care continuum. PAQs using this approach need to put the support structures in place to foster a high level of accountability.

But PAQs will need more than guidelines and triage. They also need educators who can teach patients to perform self-triage. For example, practices can create support services such as an illness evaluation site on the Internet to help parents determine whether their child has a problem such as diabetes.

One challenge of the new practice of medicine is encouraging patients and parents to use the education that the practice provides. Support services are needed to create new patient expectations. Fostering a learning environment and encouraging patients to incorporate self-care routines requires a solid plan, new employees, and the ability to measure impact. Most practices lack this type of infrastructure unless they are committed to the new practice of medicine. This type of PAQ infrastructure will become more common as rewards for building practice improvement, efficiency, and effectiveness result in shared rewards for physicians.

### Involving Patients in Care

The PAQ's success depends on physicians' including educated patients in the decisions regarding their care. According to DSM literature, educated patients can improve their own clinical outcomes. Multiple studies have shown that patients can make a prudent decision as to whether they are in a true emergency situation as long as they have education (Boulet, 1998, p. 91). The perception of an emergency by the patient appears to be based on their expectations and knowledge base. Education can contribute to the patient's knowledge base and create different expectations of medical care. Patient education also results in different outcomes, including improved patient satisfaction.

Just as patient education can be an effective management tool, every step of medical care can be maximized with an educational strategy and a specific curriculum. In the office setting, best care happens when the patient knows what to do and what to expect from care. Patient education begins with management protocols that include telephone scheduling and support, and continues across the continuum of care to the most specialized medical services provided.

As new best care strategies are considered, structures should be put in place that allow patients to make the ultimate decision about their care. The PAQ implements the care protocols to improve health, but the patient decides how or whether they fit into the PAQ philosophy. For example, the convenience and speed of care provided by lower-level ancillary care providers may actually improve satisfaction. However, the patient may feel best care is to see the physician even when a midlevel licensed provider would be sufficient. In this case, the patient's request would be met to maintain satisfaction. As another example, pap smears and annual exams for women cost less using nurse practitioners and they can be performed less frequently in low-risk patients (Amschler, 1983, p. 42). But patients have to decide whether they are comfortable with this protocol. Best care means that patients remain the final decision makers on these issues. Patient education provides the solution. The PAQ must try to establish expectations, but patients must feel they have a choice and that all of their options are appropriate.

With patient education, new expectations, and high satisfaction, the PAQ can achieve success in any environment. The PAQ recognizes that satisfied patients will return to the practice and recommend the practice to others. A good reputation is critical to every physician, so patient dissatisfaction is important to track. In addition to conducting surveys that ask whether any of the care was inadequate, the triage nurse conducts an exit interview to target serious problems when a patient leaves the practice. The results are put into a confidential report for each of the physicians in the PAQ.

Frequently it is the dissatisfied patient that helps the practice target improvements. Once problems are recognized, the PAQ systematically eliminates them after peer discussion and agreement on an action plan for change.

Patient compliance with recommendations is used to measure the impact of education; these results are connected directly to clinical and financial success. Patient satisfaction data often have no correlation with the technical quality measures of medical care, but they are a very real indicator of whether patients are happy with the PAQ model of care.

The CPI principles (described in Chapter Five) should be used to prove that the quality of care at the practice level is improving as costs are reduced. If patient involvement, satisfaction, and access can also be maintained, this new model will transform the practice.

### Achieving Optimal Utilization of Resources

As PAQs become more mature they change their operational structure considerably. Not only is there a melding of patients' needs with a proper level of medical services, but the PAQs also ensure that there is a balance between service provided and resources utilized.

All levels of the office practice must be addressed. For example, patient-centered care focuses on the resolution of illness and the benefits of prevention. To manage the continuum of care, resource utilization is allocated based on the potential for achieving prevention in addition to better medical outcomes. The physician is assumed to have the highest level of diagnosis and treatment skills. The physician teaches lower level clinical skills to all of the ancillary providers. Physician assistants, graduate nurses, therapists, and other patient assistants help the patient take on new (but safe) patient care responsibility. Through this chain of education, the PAQ physicians can trust the ancillary providers to manage that portion of care that does not require the physician. Each member of the PAQ and each employee learns to operate within a continuum of triage, treatment, and education by protocol. All of the results are measured, and improved performance is formally tracked.

Even if the patient requires hospitalization, the PAQ remains the focus for organizing medical care. The medical practice creates an expectation in patients that all medical care needs can be assessed and resolved by the PAQ as their central source of education and support. This is the case even when care is extended to the home and other community sites.

The new practice of medicine asks that each clinical and educational professional involved in care achieve efficiencies. For instance, the patient's first contact with the medical system is usually by telephone. The PAQ needs more than the typical receptionist answering the phone. This triage professional must be clinically trained to recognize the severity of the patient's problems. They must also convey empathy and caring for the patients in addition to determining their clinical needs. This new practice receptionist is also skilled at partnering with the other providers in follow-up to the first wave of triage. This first clinical interaction sets the tone for the entire medical experience. To perfect this support role, the receptionist must learn from the physicians. Physicians must provide feedback to the receptionist about providing care. In the past this position was filled by the most unskilled employee on the payroll. Now it is clear that the resources spent here become an investment in success. A smooth start always improves the medical management that follows.

*Creating Efficiency*

Innovation is one of the hallmarks of the new practice of medicine. For example, physicians might consider keeping their offices open late, since rent is paid 24 hours per day. To be efficient, the practice hires employees who will work hours convenient to the patient, both before and after regular working hours. With extended hours, patients do not need to take time off work to see their health care provider. But the PAQ should be careful to track patient satisfaction with changes, and weigh this against increased efficiency and cost. Because the PAQ values information, they will need a budget for cost accounting and clinical data management to track the effect of major decisions.

For example, PAQs analyze how the resources allocated to cover the cost of physician time compare to generated revenue. The profit per unit of physician time providing care is another useful calculation. This profit potential is calculated for in-office income generation as compared to hospital income generation. A primary care PAQ may discover that they lose money with inpatient care because of time spent sorting through hospital bureaucracies and traveling to the hospital. Calculating this cost usually shows that there is an economic loss for seeing a single hospitalized patient from one practice. As a result, the PAQ may join with other PAQs and pay a hospitalist to see all hospitalized patients. Typically, this cost is less than the revenue set aside to pay for this type of care. These hospital-based physicians are efficient because of their location and high volume. These specialists free the PAQ physicians to see patients in their own high-volume arena—the office. The key to keeping this type of new clinical process profitable is to maintain the measurement of specific outcomes and cost. This can usually be managed by the partnership's information office, described in Chapter Nine.

Laboratory services also provide a good example of how PAQs manage resource utilization. Although most small offices perform simple laboratory services, they usually have not investigated whether or not this service is cost effective. If a commercial laboratory can perform an automated CBC for $3.50, the small office must achieve the same efficiency or they should consider contracting these services out. Although patient convenience and quick results are also important considerations, the PAQ must consider these costs carefully as they are at risk for the financial outcome. After analyzing nurse time, instrument calibration, technician time, and supplies, most practices discover that they are losing money with a small-volume lab service. Even if contracting these services out will save money, this benefit must be weighed against patient satisfaction and diagnostic success.

*The Physician's Time*

Currently, there is approximately one ancillary provider for every nine physicians in practice in the United States (Cochrane, 1994). Organizations that have been pathfinders in the quest for aligned incentives (such as Friendly Hills in California) created very successful models of outpatient management by using a much lower ratio of physician to ancillary provider (Barnett, 1994, p. 66). Hiring these ancillary personnel as employees can increase physician income. One ancillary provider for every two or three physicians is an efficient ratio for most PAQs as long as computer decision support is tied to simple protocols. This means that the economic resources once reserved for physicians will be used to support a mix of providers.

Because physicians constitute the most expensive part of the care continuum, the physician's time is reserved for educating the ancillary provider and directing medical care. Surgeons' time is therefore most efficiently utilized in the operating room. Utilizing primary care support before and after surgery, the practice can exploit the physician's technical skills and maximize the physician's time to the benefit of the PAQ.

*Physician as Manager*

Optimal utilization of resources requires the physician to delegate appropriate responsibility to all the other office-based providers. This responsibility is one that many physicians have never considered. Every member of the care team will need basic management skills to maximize their ability to achieve efficiency and effectiveness in support of the physicians' ultimate medical care. This will require interdependence among all the members of the care team (this is covered in Chapter Six). To coordinate services throughout the group, physicians are utilized only in cases where the clinical diagnosis and potential treatment are uncertain. Other members of the care group can provide the remaining straightforward care and education under protocol. Because they are legally responsible for outcomes, physicians must manage personnel and supervise all this care. The physicians within PAQs find they have more time to continuously improve medical skills and to practice hands-on medical care if they are better managers.

### Providing Data Support for Clinical Decision Making

Consumer and payer groups are already measuring who the most cost-efficient providers of key services are. For instance, some third-party payers use C-section rates as a basis for contracting (Stafford, 1990). If they want the third-party contracts and a good reputation among patients, PAQ physicians need to track cost, sort out complex diagnostic possibilities, and devise treatment plans that are unique to each PAQ.

Cost accounting office-based medical services are essential to the new practices if they are to make data-driven decisions. The new practice must be able to calculate which employees are the most cost effective at providing preventive health care counseling, doing well-examinations, delivering telephone advice, sorting through a complex diagnosis, and providing inpatient care. Unit-based cost accounting measures efficiency, whereas clinical indicators determine the effectiveness of each provider. The PAQ maximizes efficiency of resources by tracking a provider's utilization and by assigning the appropriate skill-level provider to resolve specific clinical or educational issues. The provider's time can be calculated as a specific dollar amount per hour, and the real cost of an average encounter can be calculated for each visit. The questions of who gets care, where, when, at what cost, and with what outcomes are constantly being reevaluated by the new practice.

### Data: The Focus of Success

The PAQ's primary advantage over other practices is that they link data-specific strategies for improvement. The strategy for improving the efficiency of medical care is based on the fact that the outcome for most medical care is known prior to instituting therapy. Variation in the method used to achieve the expected outcome is what interests the PAQ. Most problems with inefficiency and quality result from the mistaken belief that wide variations in care are acceptable, even though they achieve the same outcome. A small PAQ can change from this faulty line of reasoning and implement consistent care by using data collection and benchmarking as the foundation.

When several PAQs are linked together, they can agree to follow the evidence of best practice until a new best practice can be achieved across an increasing number of providers. With a cooperative commitment, PAQs can share data and are motivated by each other's results. The economic success of one PAQ inspires less successful PAQs to duplicate improvements with the help of an information office (CIMCO).

PAQ physicians understand that providing the proper medical care is often linked to the consistent initiation of specific care steps within the delivery process. They examine variability at each key process step to improve overall outcomes. For example, if fever is the symptom that prompts the patient to consider medical care, the variability in specific provider response to that symptom is measured. This allows the practice to determine which response is the most efficient and to implement it throughout the PAQ.

All assumptions made by the PAQ need to be either proved or disproved. When a call is made to the physician, the patient is indicating that the information they possess is inadequate to respond to the problem they have encountered. Recognizing this, the practice can determine whether home information programs, either through triage nurses or formal education, are adequate to decrease unnecessary visits without causing harm to the patient.

*Integrating the Facts*

Technology can help the PAQ form a truly integrated office record, but the PAQs using paper records cannot wait for automation. If a computerized medical record does not exist, the PAQ should use

spreadsheets and coded data-collection tools that allow the tracking of clinical improvement. (A simple example was given for
asthma in the last chapter.) Although an interactive database can
be built on a desktop computer to track care for chronically ill
patients, a more common approach is to partner with a hospital or
health system willing to provide this type of tracking for aligned
PAQs. For example, one PAQ wanted to know the frequency of
seizures among patients on chronic seizure medications and whether
these seizures had occurred because of inadequate anticonvulsant
levels or because the patient's disease was worsening. Only by reviewing the frequencies of anticonvulsant medications, doses, and
compliance could new care tracks be devised. Even though these
data were collected on paper via a coded data sheet, the amount of
information was small enough that it could be loaded onto a personal computer prospectively for ongoing analysis.

For the sake of reimbursement, it was important for this PAQ to
prove they cared for a greater proportion of ill patients than other
practices. To create visible fairness, they needed more revenue per
member per month (pm pm), so they used data to track general acuity of illness in their patients. These data were then compared to
the general population. The PAQ focused on severity stratification
when they suspected that their patients really were sicker than those
in the average practice.

PAQs focus on data management as a key to documenting success or failure not only with treatment protocols, but also with the
goal of providing efficient care. The challenge has been to create a
universal format for data entry and reporting that is as widely
accepted as the SOAP (subjective, objective, assessment, plan)
methodology for physician progress notes. Sharing a uniform type
of electronic reporting tool aids communication just as SOAP notes
have for years. Uniform reporting also prevents PAQs from rein-
venting the wheel with each practice. Figure 11.1 shows a typical
PAQ summary report. The level of detail behind the report varies
based on the available data and goals of the PAQ. This type of

**Figure 11.1. Sample of High-Level Summary for Working Physician Group.**

---

**Success at a Glance Evidence**
*Confidential Summary Report of the Practice July '98*

For: Working Physicians Group Code 288896
Re: Personal Data

---

| Work Group Effectiveness | | |
|---|---|---|
| Total Revenue | $1,380,000 | |
| Total Expenses | $855,600 | |
| Contribution Margin | 38% | |
| **Work Group Productivity** | | |
| Number of Visits per Physician | 5,263 | |
| Percentage of Referrals out of System | 10.5% | ☆ |
| **Patient Satisfaction** | | |
| Number Surveyed | 3,470 | |
| Patient Satisfaction | 92% | |
| Perception of Access | 95% | |
| **Clinical Achievement** | | |
| Percentage of Monthly Clinical Improvement Goals Achieved | 80% | |
| Percentage of Monthly Financial Goals Achieved | 76% | |
| Cost Savings | $42,365 | |
| Incentive Bonus | $11,201 | |

☆ = significant trend exists in component of this group.

The *star* indicates that a significant trend exists in a component of this group.

report makes prospective data comparisons of revenue, patient volume, improvement goals, referrals, and savings much easier.

*Special Considerations of Shared Risk*

A PAQ using reimbursement based on capitation must show that patients seen within the office setting actually need the level of service they receive. An office-based survey linked to illness severity determines whether screening programs are appropriate and ensures that severely ill patients receive proper care.

Likewise, PAQs can determine whether telephone triage is successful by examining emergency room records for patient visits within two days of a telephone call. If the triage person felt the visit to the ER was unnecessary, a retrospective examination of the appropriateness of advice based on the future course of the illness indicates whether triage protocols are indeed working. But these types of studies take time and resources. The PAQs justify the cost of overall planning and data management by proving that the effort saves more money for the practice than it costs to put in place.

## Providing Best Patient Care

Finding best patient care within the PAQ necessitates a broader view of what is appropriate than was previously assumed. To influence the continuum of health care, efficient office management focuses on preventive health and sustained recovery as well as illness. PAQs understand that the majority of illnesses are not overly complex and that preventive health care is often a very effective way to prevent unnecessary illness. Testing this assumption via data management will probably prove that less care is part of the new definition of best care. By tracking patient satisfaction and the perception of access, the PAQ can also see whether this definition of best care aligns with what the patient wants.

Matching the need for services with the correct provider has resulted in an evolving role for nurses. Nursing services are a principle focus of resource utilization in managing the continuum of care. The choice of how to use nursing experience is highly prac-tice-dependent, but one observation can be made categorically: The skills necessary to succeed in the office setting are much different from those in the hospital setting. A detailed analysis of office-based nursing services reveal that most services, especially those provided in the primary care setting, do not require an RN level of nursing skill. Although the proper allocation of nursing services is para-mount to financial success, it should not compromise the goal of achieving best care.

Many practices employ medical assistants in formal team roles to decrease the need for registered nurses. Policies, protocols, and tracking of accountability replace mistaken assumptions about skills that have never been measured.

However, specialty practices are more likely to need specially trained graduate-level clinicians as ancillary providers to ensure quality. Office education clarifies the appropriate clinical role of physician extenders and is based on a teamwide commitment to im-provement strategies. As long as the physicians are committed to teamwork, the additional providers will be accepted. But the wise PAQ will have more physicians than extenders. This way, the med-ical community is more likely to accept that the PAQ is providing appropriate care, especially once the practice becomes more prof-itable than its peers. The real proof of "best care" is in the data col-lected by peers and regulators. The comparative data need to show that the practice is providing excellent care. The physicians create the accountability for clinical improvements that build the reputa-tion of the PAQ. Successful PAQs become the benchmark for new expectations for care.

Extenders' use of protocols also needs to be measured. The per-centage of protocol utilization can be tracked regularly to ensure learning and high-quality results. Cross-training extenders can help improve protocol utilization. Many graduate-level nursing programs and allied health professional training programs already provide cross-training for students. These professionals are able to provide numerous functions within these new office practice settings. For example, a PAQ performing intermittent radiology services may employ a practical rather than certified radiology technician and refer out more complicated radiology studies. Some simple studies can even be read by radiologists over the Internet, thus adding speed, accuracy, and cost effectiveness. This type of improvement strategy should be based on the physicians' experience and comfort at interpreting radiographs. Whatever the decision, best care will follow a practice management protocol and the results will need to be measured.

An example of delegation of accountability to achieve best care can be seen in obstetrics. The nurse midwife is a special type of physician extender. Historically, this graduate-level nurse is the oldest midlevel provider. Since the delivery of most babies remains a routine process, the midwife is a good provider for this care. But the midwife must have the skills to recognize difficulties that require more specialized care before problems develop. If difficulties arise, the physician's diagnostic and problem-resolution skills are needed. For best care, the midwife must consult the physician at the first sign of trouble. If the problem progresses, the physician's diagnostic skills are coupled with operative skills, and a Cesarean section can be performed.

PAQs are broadening the use of physician extenders to support many specialty services because these extenders are not only cost effective but also improve clinical outcomes and patient satisfaction in some cases (Holzman and others, 1994, p. 636).

Use of physician extenders changes the physician's role significantly. As more care is delivered by midlevel providers, the physician's role will shift to provide only high-risk care to patients with a higher severity of illness; as a result, the physicians' job will get harder. PAQs must align incentives that provide a greater reward for the physician's new, more challenging role.

### Evaluating Clinical Improvements

The clinical and fiscal accounting that records improvement at the practice level defines the best value or quality of care. This combination of outcome per cost determines the design of care within a PAQ. PAQs view CPI as a means to accurately manage clinical process steps tied to financial analysis in much the same way that business views production control as a time-tested principle. PAQs that use CPI are able to improve medical care and create savings in the outpatient setting. Consumers want value in health care, so health care systems must concentrate on outpatient quality. This parallels the current focus on hospital improvements. PAQs are preparing for this shift by requiring office-based CPI accountability.

Many physicians have not seen the improvement trends that are possible because they don't have a partner committed to helping them succeed in using data. In the old practice monitoring was limited to the data being collected by HMOs or hospital report cards. And the information collected usually was no more than utilization and broad morbidity and mortality reports. Their data were also based on retrospective inpatient chart reviews of face sheet data with all their inaccuracies and inherent delay.

The PAQ does not measure everything. They only analyze the key indicators needed to prove that their CPI and DSM projects are on track. They follow the project management methods previously described in Chapters Five, Nine, and Ten to ensure that they are getting the facts. By staying focused, they motivate implementation of best practices across the variety of providers within the PAQ.

Quality improvement strategies within the PAQs can also include operational indicators. The number of patients seen in the office when telephone advice would have been sufficient is a key question in quality improvement. The PAQ needs to know how many patients request hospital admission through the ER within twenty-four hours of a failed office evaluation, how may patients receive a new diagnosis when they are seen in the ER, and how often this new problem indicates that the previous diagnosis and plan were in error. As facts are used to answer these questions, they create a significant strategic advantage for the new health care partnerships.

## Operating the Practice Accountable for Quality

The experience of Phoenix Pediatrics offers a good working example of how to operate a PAQ. As President Tom Barela, M.D., describes his experiences it is clear that this group recognized the power of aligned incentives, high-quality care, and cooperative patient management to provide a medical home for their pediatric patients. Phoenix Pediatrics negotiated a direct contract with the Arizona Medicaid HMO, Access, to share risk and reward for the cost and quality of management of this very sick population. Because their contract created aligned incentives, they were able to put the PAQ principles into operation at the point of delivering care.

As Phoenix Pediatrics shifted from FFS to shared risk and potential reward, they used many of the PAQ principles. They used best care protocols, the services of pediatric medical assistants, a cross-trained medical assistant/practical radiology technician, registered nurses, and graduate-level nurse clinicians. The services and expertise of each of these professionals were blended with that of a physician partner. Through this approach they achieved high performance while offering optimal support services. Since most office-based services are not highly intensive, only one RN was on duty per shift. Although often providing routine lower level services, that nurse was also available for higher-level interactions with physicians and other providers in the office. With this strategy, the RN level of skill was made available with the specific goal of allowing the practice to extend the nurse's ability with other lower cost medical assistants.

At Phoenix Pediatrics, nursing services were an understood and analyzed cost to the practice. Although necessary for hospital-based services, registered nurse training was viewed as a luxury in the outpatient office setting by this practice. These higher-level nursing skills were maximized by allocating them to the nursing pool at specific times of the day. The same approach was used with radiology and lab services. They understood that these services did not need to be provided continuously during the workday, so the services were limited to a specific schedule.

Under the PAQ model, these ancillary providers must follow protocols that support the continuum of care outlined by the practice. The ongoing challenge for Phoenix Pediatrics became properly assessing and utilizing all of the personnel, in concert with the physicians, to achieve the necessary quality and efficiencies that defined the success of the practice. By applying this to the delivery of best care, they created optimal utilization.

All of the providers of medical services and education within the practice needed the same quality and cost mindset. This included proper use of the high-end ancillary providers such as clinical nurse practitioners, physician assistants, and nurse educators. Even in this high-risk pediatric practice, 70 to 80 percent of medical care was found to be routine and could be provided by someone other than a physician.

By training graduate-level nurses to make routine diagnoses and to recognize abnormalities along a diagnostic protocol, Phoenix Pediatrics created a safe and very cost-effective management model within the specialty services and primary care services of the practice. Though managing wellness and risk prevention were seen as valuable, the most important goal of this practice was disease state management. Implementation of best care was defined as improved clinical outcomes that demonstrated a critical contribution to the patient's health. Under this model, when patients needed less care it improved the practice's bottom line. Consequently, this measurement took on a new meaning.

After the patients had been funneled to the physician through triage, recognizing the remaining diagnostic dilemmas was the central responsibility and contribution of the physician. Physicians were held accountable for the highest risk aspects of care, and were therefore the most expensive part of the treatment team. Phoenix Pediatrics recognized that they could not afford to waste anyone's time, most especially the physicians'.

Patients and providers began to share responsibility for care to improve outcomes while lowering costs as part of the partnership's commitment to high-performance teamwork. The parents of chronically ill patients began a unique educational process that helped them assume new responsibility to comanage their children's care. This education helped the parents realize that lifestyle choices were affecting the conditions of their children. With education, the families became more willing participants in prevention. The operational PAQ principle was to involve the patient and family in care one at a time. This strategy created the greatest influence on the new partnership's goal to improve care. For example, a problem such as smoking took on new implications. The parents of an asthmatic child were aided in their own efforts to stop smoking for the sake of the child. The result was fewer hospitalizations for the child and direct savings in which the practice shared.

Another example of how the PAQ managed minor health issues can be seen in how this group of pediatricians cared for the common cold. The physicians first asked, "How many times do we treat colds with antibiotics?" To answer this question, they needed to use the PAQ principle of measurement. The data indicated wide variation, with no apparent complications in those patients who were not treated with antibiotics. The group reviewed the data in a peer discussion as part of their commitment to the PAQ principle of reaching best care through fact-based clinical decisions. They concluded that most colds were viral and did not respond to antibiotics. They also discovered that some physicians had created an unwarranted expectation on the part of the parent to receive antibiotics, even though there was no real need for the prescription. This practice pattern poses an even bigger problem in locations where access to physicians is limited. For example, in some rural areas an antibiotic is prescribed by phone to keep the family from making a long trip to see the physician. The analysis that Phoenix Pediatrics put in place tracked the cost of care for this nonmedical health issue. They also reviewed the actual clinical outcomes prospectively from that point forward. Because all of these patients got well no matter what the care, it was clear that wide cost variation between providers was not going to help the practice grow.

These physicians recognized that minor illnesses often do not require physician input for diagnosis or treatment. Their study of the common cold became a good focus for operationalizing most of the PAQ principles within the practice. They were working under aligned incentives and they had support services in place. First, they used triage and education to decrease the requests for treatment. Cost-effectiveness calculations required measurement and accounting for the employee time needed to provide these services. This was weighed against ER and office visit costs that had occurred in this population over the previous year. Because this practice was under contract to share risk, they were rewarded economically for their success even after the cost of triage and education was considered.

The most important question that continues to face this practice is, "Which other minor complaints do not need medical treatment?" Answering this question by using triage protocols, education, and outcomes measures day after day will provide the answer.

This chapter detailed the steps needed to operationalize the office practice capable of driving the success of the new health care partnerships. In the next chapter, the inevitable influence of business is addressed from the context of needed support and partnership within the new practice of medicine. New business relationships have the potential to implement even greater efficiencies in hospital and office-based care.

# 12

# Partnering with Business
## A Competitive Strategy or a Survival Necessity

The last chapter delineated the requirements for a physician practice to succeed in the new era. The concept of small groups of physicians working together was seen as the only practical method to ensure accountability for quality.

The ultimate success of the new practice of medicine requires cooperation and support from business, although many physicians have trouble believing this assumption. Rather than partnering with businesses and hospitals directly to create their long-term success, these short-sighted physicians are creating independent groups and hoping to control their short-term fee-for-service reimbursement contracts. Partnering with businesses provides a great opportunity for the new practice of medicine because businesses across the country have targeted the reduction of health care costs as a key solution to their economic stress. In addition, businesses know that a healthy employee is a productive employee. By replacing control with cooperation (Chapter Six), practices can apply high-performance cooperative models to the workplace.

Some businesses have already started to use the strategy described in this chapter. They are partnering with physicians and hospitals and avoiding the third-party payer through contracts with physician hospital organizations (PHOs), preferred provider organizations (PPOs), managed care organizations (MCOs), and provider-owned HMOs. Armed with the partnership philosophy described in this book, these businesses are beginning to collaborate. Their prime targets for partnering are physicians, hospitals, and outpatient organizations already in a health care partnership dedicated to building a healthy community, including the workforce.

Not all businesses are committed to cooperation and they continue to rely on pure cost cutting. This short-term strategy will lead to rationing as unaligned practices are forced to accept unrealistic contracts rather than risk losing patients. These two approaches, cooperation and rationing, are actually in opposition. Businesses often believe that the only way to buy good care is to force the cost of the providers down. They fail to see the resistance they are creating by forcing compliance with their guidelines and report cards. In an effort to select those who achieve the lowest cost care, they are harming their physician partners. Business purchasers of care who force their contracted providers to ignore quality issues will also lose in the long run. Until recently providers and purchasers have been able to claim that all care was good care, so purchasers drove costs down through seeking deeper discounts. Providers who continue to try to win contracts solely on cost will not fare well in the error-rate statistics as the measurements become more sophisticated. Increasing errors, such as delay to treat or failure to diagnosis, will hurt these practices and patients. The National Committee for Quality Accreditation (NCQA), Joint Commission on Accreditation of Healthcare Organizations (JCAHO), and the National Patient Safety Foundation are likely to call these predictable compromises negligence.

The new health care partnerships that embrace business can use the PAQ model (Chapter Eleven), the CIMCO support structure (Chapter Nine), and all six dimensions of physician leadership (Chapters Three through Eight) to oppose cost-based rationing. The new practice goal is to prove that cooperation can provide businesses with a strategic advantage because it improves health as it lowers cost. Businesses want to achieve the lowest costs but will not knowingly encourage dangerous care in their efforts to cut costs.

The physicians who will change care based on cost alone with little attention to clinical data are becoming visible to the purchasers of care. Driven by fear and a need to keep patients, physicians are accepting deeper and deeper discounts. They are attempting to survive under the old rules while the purchaser of their care reaps the benefits of lower cost. While businesses save money, participating physicians' incomes have hit a new low and patient injuries are becoming statistically significant (Charles and others, 1992). An alternative strategy is to encourage businesses to formally partner and to build enough cooperation to implement the new practice of medicine.

## The Benefits for Business

By using new health care partnerships as a springboard and the strategy and tactics described in previous chapters as the tools for change, there is a clear opportunity for business partners who want to participate in the new health care partnerships. Businesses allied to the new health partnership can provide better care for their employees. This becomes an ethically grounded force that draws business and providers together under a common vision. Together, they can document best value care and visible fairness through aligned incentives for aggressive disease state management and illness prevention. As true partners, the businesses that join the new health care partnerships actually strengthen their workforce through better care.

Businesses can use contracts to describe reimbursement for the care that they are purchasing. The information that defines success of the partnership can then be linked to the business to fulfill the contract. The potential to lower overall cost varies greatly, depending on volume, ability to take on risk, and the age of the patients. However, the savings described earlier now benefit the business in an agreed-upon formula. This strategy requires data and accurate projections of savings. These projections are based on an assessment of the business employee demographics, so a cooperative open-sharing of data should be established prior to contracting the relationship. Businesses that are seeking this type of health care relationship are usually willing to provide access to summary data on previous cost of care for employees.

There will be fewer practicing physicians, fewer hospital beds, more allied health providers, more home care organizations, and a much lower cost of care in the coming years. As a rule, businesses believe that the cost of care will come down, so physicians should put a strategy in place that takes this assumption into account. The first step for the partnership is more financial forecasting. If financial projections cannot be made because of a lack of knowledge or data, the strategy to partner with businesses may be unsound.

By maintaining their integrity and placing the needs of their patients first and foremost, physicians can safely partner with other physicians to achieve the necessary volume for attracting business allies. Together, these expanded partnerships can forecast and then manage their future. In addition, physicians committed to the new partnerships need to reassure themselves that their success does not harm their peers.

## Information Sets the Rules

The environment for a health care business partnership has been evolving over the past twenty years, and although each location will have its own terrain to negotiate, several rules of the game are clearly in place. These rules are not all economic. In 1975, the Supreme Court ruled that the profession of medicine was subject to the Federal antitrust law and could no longer prohibit open competition among its physicians (Bergthold, 1990, p. 20). This ruling led to open comparisons of physicians, advertising, and the opportunity for businesses to purchase medical care based on cost information.

By the 1970s the third party began to administer the purchase of care and track the delivery for the purpose of billing. These third-party businesses thrived by selling insurance to other businesses and the public. Under this system, catastrophic illness could be paid for by spreading the individual burden of these extreme costs to the entire membership.

The majority of clinical outcomes were not actually measured because computers were not used for this purpose. Third-party businesses did not have the technological tools and there was a general belief that all medical care was excellent. Since all care was viewed as best care, it made perfect sense for businesses to purchase care like any other defined commodity. After all, credentials were required, physicians were well educated, and the national and state medical societies were in place to ensure quality. Peer review organizations (PROs) had been formed state by state to verify that providers with serious quality problems would not go unrecognized. However, without information about qualitative differences in care, buying medical care seemed as straightforward as buying sowbelly or corn on a commodity exchange. It was during this era that businesses established rules for dealing with the health care industry.

RULE 1: *Assuming all care is of the same quality, businesses should buy the lowest cost care from whomever can administer and deliver the care.*

This rule is based on the old assumptions that were being made in the 1970s that all care was best care, and that we would never be able to differentiate quality. Even though that has changed with the ability to process data, many people still erroneously believe that medicine is an art and cannot be measured. Dealing with businesses that operate under this assumption is a real disadvantage to any new integrated systems.

### The Move to Clinical and Cost Measurement

In 1971, HMOs adopted a national health strategy to lower the cost of care. They were able to provide care for less, but they did not have the outcome data to explain how they were managing it. Over the next ten years the concept of small area analysis and comparison of medical practice variation in similar communities was developed (Wennberg and others, 1973, pp. 1102–1108). John Wennberg pioneered the effort in 1973, and the Maine Medical Assessment Foundation expanded his work well into the 1990s and proved that wide variation in clinical practice is very real (Wennberg, 1999, pp. 52–53). The Stanford Center for Health Care Research also contributed to the movement with a clinical comparison of hospitals in 1976 (Stanford Center for Health Care Research, 1976, pp. 112–127). The National Halothane study from the 1960s had shown a three-fold difference in fatalities by hospital, but it wasn't until the 1970s that data analysts began to discuss it (Moses and Mosteller, 1968, pp. 150–152).

RULE 2: *Large businesses can manage the health benefits of their employees.*

Another rule guiding businesses is that the third party payer is not a necessity when paying for care. This assumption arose from the health care environment of the 1970s. The cost of care wasn't a subject of analysis until then. In 1974, the Employee Retirement Income Security Act (ERISA) became law and gave large, self-insured corporations, who felt costs were too high, the freedom to design their own health benefit plans. This was a significant shift in business thinking. Large corporations such as Chrysler had analyzed their costs and determined that the wide variation in their highest business expense, health care, was unacceptable. To compete on a global scale with foreign car manufacturers, they decided they would only buy the services of hospitals and doctors who provided the most efficient and appropriate care.

Chrysler, with half a billion dollar health care budgets, conducted medical audits as a justification for using HMOs to cut down on costs. What the audit revealed was not only inefficiency and waste, but also clear overutilization and fraud (Califano, 1986, pp. 17–52). For the first time, large coalitions of national companies, such as Washington Business Group on Health, joined together to take control away from the health insurers. With this change in the rules, businesses had to make direct comparisons of the physicians' care, or at least the hospitals' care, to buy the right services.

RULE 3: *The difference in clinical outcomes will be measured and made public whether or not the physicians and hospitals perform the measurement.*

Until ERISA legislation, thirty-two states had laws that prohibited the use of information to clarify the differences between physicians. Once ERISA became law, the business rules changed again.

When the ERISA legislation made comparisons legal it seemed logical that these comparisons would be made public. Once this happened it would be possible for businesses to make these comparisons in an ongoing way at a very low cost.

Stories like the nine-fold difference in comparative hospital statistics on open-heart mortality were front-page news. As the 1980s unfolded, the Health Care Financing Administration (HCFA) began publishing hospital mortality rates. The press used the Federal Freedom of Information Act to obtain the information.

During this era there was a major shift in the thinking of both businesses and the public. Because of the bad press, many consumers began to suspect that some care was not actually very good. The medical community followed the lead of public health departments and responded to the public's desire to compare physicians. The medical community had its own need to know why the variations were so great. The Journal of the American Medical Association published the results of open-heart surgery in New York state in 1990. Comparison of risk-adjusted death rates showed dramatic differences by physician, and the greatest variation was seen among practitioners who did less than 100 cases per year (Hannan, 1990,

p. 2768). A year later, the press won the battle to get the names of the cardiovascular surgeons from the New York State Department of Public Health, and a front page article was published with the actual physicians' names and information about their specific performance. This event marked the beginning of a demand for accountability that forced the health care profession to shift from an unmonitored and above-suspicion profile to a comparison-driven environment.

The New York physicians are not pleased that their names and outcomes are made public information yearly, but this is unlikely to change. In fact, other states are following suit. These comparisons are likely to persist because they appear to have an effect. The level of accountability forced on the cardiovascular surgeons in New York resulted in the risk-adjusted death rate for bypass patients dropping by 40 percent. The Cardiac Surgery Reporting System (CSRS), which evolved as a result of New York's reporting efforts, is recognized as a health care reporting leader by businesses across the country. In many states, business purchasers of care use CSRS to define the best practices and providers of cardiac services. Physicians now face a new challenge: They need to be in the top half of all the publicly compared outcomes or they will be accused of being substandard.

These new reporting and comparison strategies led some to fear that physicians would simply stop performing high-risk procedures to avoid the possibility of a low rating. CSRS took that fear into consideration. They decided to use risk adjustment that over-predicts the probability of death in the severely ill (Hannan, 1990, p. 2770). Using this strategy, an average surgeon who takes higher risk patients would be more likely to get a lower than expected mortality rate. This comparison feature actually encourages the physicians to treat the high-risk patients. With this type of research base for comparison of data in place, researchers and other academics began to publish highly regarded, in-depth comparisons of clinical outcomes (Leape, 1993, p. 753).

The effect of public information and the health community's acceptance of public comparisons of clinical outcomes will completely change how a provider operates. Thousands of different businesses will use the new data comparisons to shop for health care. Providers must take these businesses' attitude and approach into account as they set their budgets and then purchase care. Some states have made it a priority to search out cost and quality information, such as the Pennsylvania Health Care Cost Containment Council, a legislated body. The Council's goal is to attach clinical outcome data to the specific physicians and hospitals that provided the care (Sessa, 1992, p. 44). The presence and accessibility of comparison data leads directly to the next rule.

RULE 4: *Business will lower their costs and encourage improved quality of care by deciding whose services to buy.*

Using comparison data, businesses in Pennsylvania learned that there was a great variability in the quality of care. Frequency of surgery in the population varied by 25 percent. In Philadelphia the hospital mortality rates after cardiovascular surgery had a three-fold difference from one facility to another. The business purchasers of care responded to this information. It had a significant impact on hospital admissions; some facilities even closed cardiac services (Schneider, 1996, p. 251).

By 1996, thirty-seven other states were collecting and publishing some type of health quality data, and they were becoming more organized through the National Association of Health Data Organizations. The effect of this type of data has been dramatic and has raised serious ethical questions. In one area, the hospital mortality rates for conditions like myocardial infarctions were eighteen times higher in the indigent patient population than they were in the affluent population (Siro, 1996, p. 30). Because this type of mortality data was attributed to individual physicians, their hospitals, and their health plans, businesses began to ask the next logical question, "Why are the variations occurring?" Health care organizations who answer, "We will never know" will lose business support. The successful new health care partnerships answer, "We are the benchmark that is statistically better than those practices that you should be comparing to us." The businesses that take advantage of this type of information believe they are getting better care. Many businesses utilize the new comparisons in an attempt to influence their employees to use specific plans that will help the bottom line and also ensure that they receive high-quality care.

RULE 5: *Those practices that can decrease cost and improve clinical outcomes internally prior to comparisons by businesses will be the most successful.*

The health care partnerships using the new practice of medicine have already proven that using data to guide medical decisions improves outcomes. If these partnerships can create a strategy that utilizes internal data to fix problems and improve outcomes prior to public comparison, they will have a distinct advantage over the competition when it comes to direct business contracts.

Businesses usually decide what care to buy based on public data, obtained primarily from Medicare, Medicaid, and insurance billing. The source is often referred to as the UB–92 sheet. Physicians who create their own quality data and manage the costs internally, with the skills and structure described as the new practice of medicine, can fix internal quality problems before they become public. The challenge for the new practice is to motivate physicians to change and put the structures for internal data comparison in place. The knowledge that they will be compared to other groups of providers in the purchasing arena is usually not enough motivation to change physicians' behavior. Physicians need to see how maintaining this data advantage will directly help their practices. The easiest route to this new awareness is through economic reward.

For example, the Minneapolis, St. Paul–based Business Health Care Action Group (BHCAG) emerged in the 1980s to define the requirements to succeed in the competition to provide care to patients of Minneapolis and St. Paul. This business coalition defined success very simply: They wanted good low-cost care based on data. Initially, much of the care in this region was still provided by groups of physicians who had not yet adapted the new practice methods described here despite businesses' reliance on data to buy care. Groups like Mayo Clinic, Allina Health System, Park Nicollet Medical Center, and Health Partners have only recently begun to use reward to guide physician's behavior. Initially some physicians within these systems felt that they were being pushed rather than invited into partnerships. Although the above organizations mounted a force that ensured data collection and improvements in the quality of hospital care that was being purchased, most physicians remained in a passive role. Many physicians resented working harder and harder for less and less, but felt powerless to have an impact. Because they had not organized their own internal data, these physicians had no strategy. They worked harder and waited for the large health care plans to report back to them what kind of care they were providing (Christianson, 1995, p. 114).

### Business Demanding Change

BHCAG was not interested in simply fixing lower fees for each service. Such efforts could force providers to increase the volume of patient care to keep incomes stable. The BHCAG wanted higher value for the dollar. To find it, they decided to do a cost benefits analysis on the care that was currently being provided. Their initial review of insurance data from Blue Cross & Blue Shield of Minnesota showed unacceptable variations in care, such as four- and five-fold variation in procedures for the same diagnosis. This level of variation in health care was not acceptable to the business members of the BHCAG.

The first response was to send out a request for proposal (RFP) to all of the area hospitals and health systems that demanded a commitment to quality improvement that was not only in writing, but could be continuously updated. It demanded evidence that improvement ideas were not only being implemented, but that they resulted in improved results, that guidelines were actually being used, and underutilization and overutilization were being evaluated and changed. They expected the health systems to do surveys of physician office practices for quality, even if the physicians did not lead the effort. They asked that procedure-specific standards be met in more than a dozen major costly procedures with specific measures of quality. The RFP insisted on open access to case volume data for each institution as well as individual providers. They demanded data on length of stay, inhospital mortality, complication rates, annual patient survival, unplanned returns to the OR/ER, and unplanned hospital readmissions for the same problem. Demanding these comparisons determined which practices would succeed because the winning practices had the best data according to the BHCAG (Millenson, 1997, p. 236).

The strategy for the new practice of medicine empowers practices to know how they compare in value before businesses conduct their own, broad, slow comparisons. Practices that find they have below average results would still have time to work smarter and remedy the problem before their poor data were exposed publicly. Once poor outcomes are made public, practices risk losing patients and access to other groups of patients. BHCAG, for instance, represented more than 10 percent of the population. The practices who fail to improve their data will be bypassed in favor of those who can document they are improving the quality and cost of care. Other business coalitions similar to BHCAG are organizing rapidly around the country. With comparisons widespread, the challenge for physicians is to get organized and begin to cooperate early enough and fast enough to lead the data race. Their future will be based on their ability to consistently improve the data created by the care they provide.

### Cannibalizing Our Own

In some areas, the competition and selective contracting process has been so subtle that physicians hardly realize that they are being reduced in number. In other areas, the competition is so overt and ugly that physicians must witness their colleagues' closing practices and dropping privileges.

For example, in San Diego, California, there is a primary care independent practice association (IPA) that contracts with HMOs at such a low rate that specialty IPAs cannot compete. Once they lose access to patients, the specialty IPA's income is inadequate to cover costs, and the business collapses. The primary care IPA then approaches the individual specialists with the best utilization data and offers them subcapitated contracts. The other specialists are left with no real options. This strategy is only possible because utilization data are publicly recorded. The high-cost utilizers are taken out of the picture. This primary care IPA is growing, but can they really be considered a success? As with any examples of extreme change, one group can become short-sighted and focus almost solely on self-interest. Sometimes they even destroy their own critical partners. This is what happens when groups of physicians compete on dollars alone. They are caught with one foot in the old medical paradigm and the other foot in the new. Without the right information and good clinical data, even full-risk contracting does not ensure success of the new practice strategy. In some areas, the health care environment is so competitive that physicians are cannibalizing their peers. In San Diego, contract-hungry practices have driven the cost down further in a marketplace already facing the lowest reimbursement in the country. The surviving practices cannot even see they are on the edge of doing harm to themselves as well as patients. These radical survival strategies will not lead to long-term success. They will not lead to the new practice of medicine.

### Helping Businesses Decide

Once it becomes common for quality data to be weighed side by side with cost, the businesses purchasing care will be naturally guided to the new practice strategy because they will have the data to prove best value. The real question that will shape the future is, "Will businesses ever buy more costly care when the alternative, although cheaper, is visibly lower quality?" The new practice of medicine will be forced to get this question out in front of businesses. When the employees are seen in the doctor's office as patients they will need to be given access to data so they can be informed enough to demand the best care. If patients can then go back to businesses as employees and influence the organization to buy quality, the new practice strategy will be complete.

In Minneapolis and St. Paul, large and small businesses are forming coalitions based on BHCAG's success. Although small businesses usually experience more difficulty leveraging enough power to negotiate the best contracts, the principles are the same. The Institute for Clinical Systems Integration (ICSI), which grew out of BHCAG, provides a good example of a medical community responding to the business pressure to "buy right" (Reinertson, 1993, p. 451). ICSI includes two HMOs (Group Health and Medical Centers Health Plan), the Mayo Clinic, Park Nicollet Medical Center, and over 2,000 affiliated physicians. This large group is attempting to use the practice principles of clinical improvement and disease state management as a gold standard. They ask that their providers' care be based on scientific evidence and follow group interpretation of the literature. Their definition of continuous improvement is that guidelines are put in place as tools to be challenged and changed, as providers define best care.

### Aligning the Incentives

ICSI has not yet achieved total success because their size prevents a clear link to the physicians' daily work. Without the PAQ concept of aligned incentives, the most efficient individual group practices could actually suffer a drop in revenue. In the past, some practices were so successful in preventing disease that they lost the volume of fee-for-service patients necessary to keep their doors open. The business plan for both the BHCAG and the large provider institutions was working fine, but without a partnership with physicians and visible fairness the model broke down. Early contracts were not structured on these principles and, as a result, some practices were punished even though they improved their patients' health.

The new practice must learn from these early mistakes. Even with the highest quality care, if a fair partnership among businesses, the hospitals, and physicians is not in place, the physicians will lose because of the way the fee-for-service contract is structured. Under fee-for-service, when physicians provide better and more efficient care to a fixed population of patients, they lose revenue.

Because the BHCAG captured the savings, they succeeded. But they knew that long-term success would require more equal partnerships with physicians. Consequently, they decided to contract directly with groups of physicians under shared risk, thus opening the door to the new practice reward systems. This single decision almost ensures that the transformation of health care delivery in the Twin Cities area will now move at an accelerated rate and be more physician-driven.

RULE 6: *Providers who can manage improvement, align incentives, and build business partnerships in the service to patients will thrive.*

The next generation of businesses will be reducing absenteeism by promoting health at the worksite as an economic strategy. They will create new data reports to demonstrate the true benefits of the care that their employees are receiving. The businesses will still be looking for the lowest cost but as outcome data become public they will need to respond to their employees' demands for best care and access to the best practices. The pressure to keep a top-quality workforce will push businesses to align with the new health care partnerships wherever physician leadership has opened this door. Businesses will be looking for best value whenever a difference in quality can be documented. Some will be driven by a profit motive, some by an effort to retain employees, but in either case the question of strategic partnerships with the new practice will dominate business planning of the future. The penetrating question for the providers will be, "How can we organize quickly enough to create the competitive advantage businesses are looking for?"

Businesses are responding to economic pressures and to both clinical and economic information that they can now more easily access. It is clear that business will play a much greater role in the transformation of health care in the near future. Most likely, they will influence the third-party payment industry to support the new health care partnerships described here. As the providers organize, they will prove to businesses that their practices can deliver better care than the competition. The last step for these new successful partnerships will be to partner with the community.

This chapter has projected a set of rules that will define success within the health care delivery system as businesses are increasingly able to access health care data. Chapter Thirteen outlines specific steps for the mature health care partnership to lead a transformative change within the community.

# 13

# Building for a Healthy Community

The last chapter explored how business has responded to the changing health care environment, specifically to health care costs and the recent access to comparative data. Collaborating with business will create significant opportunities for the new health care partnerships. This chapter provides the new health care partnerships with a structured approach, not only to influence community health but also to lead it. The method for leading community health included here is not based on theory, but on many years of practical experience. A variety of real-life examples have been added to illustrate the range of potential projects that an organized partnership can undertake.

The highest goal of the new practice of medicine is improving the overall health of the community. The concept of partnering with the community (the sixth dimension of physician leadership) is revisited here because it provides the most enduring means for improving the health and quality of life in America. The proactive behavioral change of patients, their families, payers, purchasers, and all providers within a community arena defines the boundaries of our ability to care.

## Community Health and the New Practice

As recently as twenty years ago, communities were disconnected and unable to optimize individual and community health. One of the main obstacles was the physicians' belief that care could not be administered until a manifestation of outward symptoms was in evidence. The goal of subsequent treatment was thus limited to the alleviation of specific symptoms or eradication of organ-specific disease, rather than searching for the overall root cause of the illness. Solutions such as lifestyle change or the coordination of treatment to encompass social, emotional, economic, and even spiritual factors were seldom considered. As a result, the root cause of disease would go untreated, thereby allowing new symptoms to resurface in a specific area at a later time. For example, a patient with vague symptoms of nasal congestion, difficulty swallowing, coughing, or hoarse speech might be diagnosed with chronic laryngitis and sinusitis after CAT scans and even laryngoscopy by an ear, nose, and throat (ENT) specialist. The doctor would rule out cancer of the larynx and start a treatment that might include prolonged antibiotics, steroids, and mucolytics to decrease the drainage and another CAT scan to check the progress of treatment.

But the root cause of the problem could be the patient's environment. Secondary smoking and pets could be causing allergies and mild adult asthma. Or if the individual is a teacher or a sales representative, how they form words during a long day of talking could be the root cause of their problem. A visit to a speech therapist might be the solution, but a visit to another specialist, this time a gastroenterologist, would probably lead to a different diagnosis. The gastroenterologist might diagnose the problem as esophageal reflux. This diagnosis would warrant yet another medical regimen to cure the elusive symptoms. If a benign polyp was seen on the original CAT scan for sinusitis and the symptoms persist, a doctor might suggest an operation to remove it.

The list of possible medical approaches for this problem is virtually endless, especially if any of these treatments caused a complication. As more care is provided, even more care could be required. But it might simply be that anxiety or aging is changing the patient's voice and disrupting the swallowing process slightly. By resolving difficult relationships at home or getting a better job, the patient might alleviate these symptoms. Whatever the root cause, medicine has not traditionally focused its attention here. Physicians have been rewarded for treating the symptoms over and over, but now it is necessary to move beyond this reductionist approach.

We now know that most disease is preventable, and in most cases of disease, recovery can be shortened and sustained. The research has shown that most adverse health conditions are not caused by the lack of sufficient medical technology or lack of patient access to medical professionals. The cause of most disease is a failure on the part of the patient to prevent the onset of the condition.

## Partners in the Delivery of Care

Significant improvements to community health will not be in the hands of physicians alone because the old independent relationship between organizations and individuals cannot improve a community's health in a meaningful way by using the solutions that worked in the old medicine. The solutions for improving community health are found in the relationships that are formed between all sectors of the community that affect health and quality of life. The issues of housing, crime, environment, economic development, spirituality, and education, in addition to health care, all have an influence on a population's health status. The challenge is for the new health care partnerships to harness these services for the benefit of individuals served. To do so, physicians in the new partnerships must embrace the multiple roles of integrator, coach, facilitator, health visionary, and cooperative community leader in addition to that of provider.

Within the old acute care model, not only were illnesses the access point and focus of treatment, but they were also thought to describe the entire, albeit narrow, continuum of care for the patient. Because even chronic illness was often viewed as multiple disconnected episodes of acute symptoms, physicians did not typically consider other providers in the community as part of the continuum.

Because these other providers were not included in the medical delivery system, they were not invited to make a contribution. This was especially true of nontraditional or alternative health care providers.

The new health care partnerships are committed to developing true continuums of care, uniting a broader integrated delivery system by including public and private entities in addition to medical providers. By using data management and shared economic incentives (described in earlier chapters), these new health care partners can see the value of incorporating organizations such as businesses, schools, churches, and health departments into their clinical improvement strategies.

Communities have minimized the leadership role of the physician because physicians have abdicated this role in the past. Physicians now stand at a crossroads. On the one hand, physicians must acknowledge the continuing need for research, investigational study, and improved, effective medical practice within specialized areas. On the other hand, their own success will be limited if they do not acknowledge that the traditional reductionist focus of medicine is not enough. As medical care issues, such as reimbursement, become even more complex and potential technical solutions more diverse and costly, the ability to identify the multiple root causes of illness will become a more important component of care success. Understanding the complex spheres of behavioral change will allow new patient behavior to be managed and tracked with community support.

## Coordinating Communities of Care

The new practice of medicine depends on focused, specialized medical expertise to devise a patient care plan that ensures positive outcomes. However, this aspect of care is simply one contributor to an interdependent whole that encourages the synergistic coordination of practitioner, provider, payer, promoter, employer, community, and individual. This whole system is based on the notion that optimal health has as much or more to do with social, emotional, environmental, economic, and spiritual issues as it does with the physical issues on which traditional, specialized medical paradigms have focused. The new practice strategy depends on a multifaceted developmental approach to community-directed health care delivery that actually decreases the frequency of illness while encouraging holistic wellness of the patient within society.

This new strategy goes well beyond placing public health or wellness pamphlets in physicians' offices for education. The PAQs explore the nature of the root causes behind disease. They are willing to test disease-management strategies that create motivation for behavioral change by drawing on cultural issues within communities and subcommunities. The American Society of Public Health, the Center for Disease Control, and local health departments all understand this new paradigm, yet in the past they rarely found it possible to partner with the physicians or hospital community. Public health departments are just now beginning to consider the value of becoming more involved with practicing physicians. By partnering with PAQs, public health departments can contribute their knowledge of coalition building, disease prevention, health promotion, and data collection for the underserved to the direct delivery of medical care.

The improvement of individual health and the comprehensive building of healthy communities are dependent on two critical issues: the management of health risks in a population, and the unified vision of collaborative commitment to planning for the involvement of all the critical community organizations. Through these efforts, the PAQs can select the best area for developing specific continuums of care. Furthermore, PAQs can target a population and gain the support of specific organizations in the community, one diagnosis at a time.

## Collaborative Planning for Community Partnerships

As part of the collaborative planning process, the new health care partnerships efficiently develop comprehensive plans to improve global health by using population health risk management and direct care protocols during one-on-one encounters. The goal of this effort is to use data to prove that cooperation reduces costs and improves satisfaction. By building formal community continuums of support, the new practice assures effective partnership for appropriate care, early access to patients, and increasing cost efficiency. Overall savings are achieved, and the comprehensive nature of a healthy community has a positive effect on health care delivery.

### Working Together Toward a Vision

Remember that a community, although vastly complex, is actually a system of specific interdependent parts. As with all systems, improvement is dependent on the coordination of all the parts under laws of cause and effect. No one organization or individual working alone is able to accomplish as much improvement for this system as by working together. To build a community system, physicians and all the constituent parts of what will become the healthy community need a unified and transformational vision. Each community will have its own unique vision and define the steps needed to move toward planning and action differently. Within a community that has established a driving vision for improved health through cooperation, it is possible for the involved organizations to work together simultaneously toward accomplishing that vision. In achieving this vision, a needed reassurance emerges that will sustain individuals as roles and organizations begin to change.

### Projects for Health Assessment and Improvement

Many communities are doing a comprehensive assessment of community health risks every three to four years. Usually this is funded from public health dollars. Initial measurements can be used as an internal benchmark. All improvement activities of the new practice can be gauged by the impact they have on these baselines of community health status. The physician is critical to this process once assessment moves from a wellness focus to specific disease management. Involved physicians can make a contribution by giving input to the design of research, selecting indicators, determining appropriate programmatic decisions, and determining resource allocation. If this level of physician volunteerism is lacking, the PAQs in the new partnerships can at least share data with each other to develop community health care forecasts. The practices can project what resources were required in the management of patient demand to ensure appropriate utilization. They can review their experience and design projects that justify resource allocation for appropriate innovations to be conducted within the community. The partnerships have a vested interest to do these calculations as part of their effort to find efficiency and cost savings. The PAQs find a similar motivation.

## Physician Leadership Benefits the Community

Physician leadership can be the cornerstone of community health. Physicians can be moved by the vision of community-wide cooperation to see the opportunities for success. The changes in their practice will result in long-term personal benefits, both in the delivery of health care and financially, but to reap these rewards most physicians must change. Some of the changes required for physicians to be effective from a community perspective include the following:

*Physicians become visionaries.* Developing an ability to understand trends that influence future decisions regarding patients, practice, integrated delivery systems, and community is a critical new skill. Physicians in the new practice are able to translate multiple trends by looking at focused data to guide all components of the system, including payers. As these physicians become visionaries, they advance the practice of medicine clinically and economically while ensuring financial success.

*Physicians understand managed care and capitation.* Physicians who fully understand issues of managed care and capitation can see the potential success of establishing community involvement. They realize that when a large number of chronically ill patients within the population are overusing medical care, too much time is being used and potential income lost by treating the patients. Because this overtreatment creates a significant negative impact to physicians' personal income, the emerging PAQs are motivated to develop alternative practice models through redistribution of work to other community professionals and organizations. This reduces the cost of primary care and the need for specialty care while creating a financial benefit for the PAQ. This approach also increases the physician's access to the savings that accumulate under shared-risk payments. The PAQ readily sees that developing a community network as part of the new practice collaborative is the most effective way to accomplish this economic success.

*Physicians become community leaders.* The physicians in the new practice are involved in the community. Physician alliances with community organizations are critical to community-wide holistic change. Physicians acting as chairs or co-chairs of community health project teams provide input to the clinical component of community activities. In turn, they learn where community support can improve the management of their own practice's future. Community leadership provides physicians with opportunities to embrace and direct change. The new practice will gain momentum as more physicians move from reluctant followers to leaders of change.

*Physicians broaden their definition of health and their practice of medicine.* The new physician's view of health and their own practice of medicine is expanded to include social, environmental, emotional, economic, and spiritual aspects. Both specialist and primary care physicians are beginning to recognize that they cannot personally provide enough interventions to improve all aspects of the patient's health. As an alternative to underserving the patient population, these physicians build strong partnerships with other providers and then act as facilitators and coordinators of health status improvement. These efforts are managed and accounted for within each PAQ and make a real contribution to the practice of medicine.

*Physicians become community organizers.* Physicians can provide a unique ability to manage the complexity that community organizers with multiple perspectives bring to the table to work for global health status improvement. Physician's medical training in cause-and-effect relationships, coupled with a need for detail and facts, is invaluable to what are often initially disorganized coalitions.

*Physicians empower their patients to become partners in the care process.* Patients' ability to understand their role in personal health improvement through education varies. Determining this ability is not an easy process, nor is it universally successful. The patient's denial, projection, and minimization of problems impede the improvement of personal health practices. Physicians in the new practice recognize these limitations and provide advice to the educational team that helps the patient take on a realistic role in self-care. Within the new practice, several clinics have chosen to implement lifestyle coaches to assist the patients. These visionaries are often retrained nurses and medical assistants who work hand in hand with the physicians to assist the patients in attaining their health goals, while saving the physician's valuable time. Specific prevention plans are developed to support healthy behaviors.

## Launching the New Practice of Medicine–Community Partnership

A fully integrated new medicine community system consists of at least one hospital, a group of physicians, and other care providers organized into accountable business units, community service organizations, public health, a business coalition, a payer, and, of course, the patient and family. This model places the providers in a partnership with the community. The data office, or CIMCO (as detailed in Chapter Nine), is ideally housed in this new health partnership.

The work of this new system includes determining the process for managing care, how health system resources are allocated, and how health care dollars paid by community residents should be used.

The financial goal is for the partnership to capture a greater portion of the health care dollar that is being spent by businesses and residents of the community and save it for reinvestment. The partnership through the data office is able to support savings by helping the providers manage the care of the community residents and by reducing actual demand for medical care.

## Establishing a Business to Manage the Partnership

A formal business entity, or several, can assume the responsibility for coordinating the medical care and education over the continuum of care needed by the residents of the community served. It is this integrated health care business that accepts the responsibilities and risks for managing care in the community. That means it can absorb losses, as well as distributing gains while building equity. Stop-loss insurance is purchased against the risk of catastrophic illness to ensure economic stability.

This new nonprofit business must fully integrate the activities of the new health partner system that is responsible for delivering the coordinated care needed by the residents of the community. This business within the system needs to align the use of data and rewards to support decision making and operations throughout the delivery of care, education, and feedback.

The key elements necessary for success must be strategically aligned to sustain the new business. A critical mass of paying patients is of prime importance, which means the partnership must have access to enough insured patients. Once there are enough paying patients to keep several practices (or PAQs) economically viable, the remainder of the patient population that constitute a community is added to the computations. Then coordinating the services for this entire community becomes the focus through reducing duplication and optimizing efficiency. The next step for the practice is improving medical care as coordinated with home care education and reduced patient demand. The final and most challenging element of management is the reallocation of savings and redesign of the care model.

The governance, management, and internal culture can be guided by the facts being managed by the data office. The new partnership's framework outlines the decision-making support needed to get the right information to the right people at the right time, and in a way that enables the many organizations to cooperate.

Beyond setting the direction, there is also the practical world of work to manage. Specific objectives, measures, and targets for customer performance, operational performance, internal growth, skills development, and financial analysis don't just happen, they must be planned. Formal training, based on cooperation and high performance (Chapter Six), must replace the distrust and self-interest that were a part of the paradigm of traditional medicine.

## Taking the Steps Required to Move Forward

The new community system must make some critical decisions early on, such as what group will be accountable for consistent direction and leadership when it comes to governing, managing, and developing the infrastructure for the partnership. This leadership or management group is critical. Everyone involved with the new partnership will be required to commit to supporting this leadership group, so data reporting and communication will be critical. The partnership will also need to allocate resources on a systemwide rather than individual-provider basis to align performance with partnership goals. This requires a commitment to agreed-upon compensation incentives that do not change midstream. The following suggested steps to get the community partnership going can be used as a checklist to ensure movement and success. The method to achieve each step will vary in each community; however, each time an item is checked off, progress is being made.

- Develop a core of at least thirty physicians (or all of those in a smaller community) who are philosophically committed to the vision and engaged in providing medical expertise as a contribution to the larger partnership. Keep a record of their names and practice locations.

- Establish the organizational framework for the partnership. This step will vary in each community and will require legal advice.

- Gather market and performance information from which to begin development and implementation of the core functional processes. List the key indicators of success. If success cannot be projected after a market analysis, then more developmental work is needed prior to launching the partnership.

- Set up the financial and clinical tracking of data (described in Chapter Nine) that is capable of ensuring success in FFS but is also capable of accounting for success or failure when risk is shared.

- Develop executive support for managing and accounting within the PAQ model (described in Chapter Eleven).

- Monitor the PAQ's clinical success as the community assists in supporting prevention and disease state management. Document the PAQ's successes as the community partnership grows.

- Clarify that the governance of the new health care partnership is committed to the new practice concepts described here. That means, at the very least, the system has the ability to assist the PAQ to achieve a financial benefit for participating in cooperation.

*Checkpoint:* If you are unable to reach this point, continue to build and implement the concepts that were outlined in Chapters Three through Seven before moving to this final dimension of the transformation. Once you have built this level of physician commitment and reward, you are ready to continue your effort.

- Next your new partnership can expand its organizational framework to include specific community projects. The data office (described in Chapter Nine) needs to accept community-generated data formally. The hospital and physician leadership is integrated into an administrative support structure that provides a hub for operations that will reach into the community.

- Market information and data on patient need is then used to create the feasibility analysis for a financially sound strategy to improve performance by achieving a small but rapid success.

- The next step is implementation of an improvement method (similar to the one described in Chapter Five). The function of the data office, the steering committee, and the key interfaces for provider and community organizational cooperation are now tested.

- As success occurs it needs to be communicated back to those who made it happen, as well as to the community being served.

- Public awareness must now take on a more central role; that is, more formal communication efforts will need to be implemented. This requires a clear priority to communicate the implementation of high-profile public projects as well as measurement of the clinical improvements and dollars saved.

- Additional PAQs and more community support are added as more community members switch providers to get their care within the new health care partnership.

- Finally, a network evolves. Clinical performance improvement goals are broadened by following the successes of other community support efforts as each gets more organized. These successes can be shared on the Internet. For example, the website www.newpracticemed.com has been established by MRM as a networking and learning environment to facilitate this type of transformation. VHA and other organizations are doing the same.

## The New Health Care Partnerships "Walk the Talk"

The new partnerships believe in cooperation and learning because of their focus on visible fairness. They develop clinical and financial policies and procedures that are realistic and achievable; that is, procedures that can be implemented and are based on medical principles, health, education, and an understanding of community support. The partnerships remain committed to developing a health-centered environment that encourages the health of the providers and volunteers as well as of patients.

Applying this philosophy to the entire community presents numerous challenges but also opportunities. The above list shows the most significant steps that need to be taken to achieve success. The new competencies needed to meet these challenges require education and training. Success of the community partnership can be approached as one would plan to add any new set of clinical skills. The training is achieved and then the skill is used in practice. The difference is that the results of using these new organization and management skills will affect the operational improvement of the practice rather than resolution of a specific illness. In the past, physicians have not placed much value on the business operation of their practice. Yet in the current health care climate, business success or failure is determined by the physician's ability to make a contribution. Both business acumen and medical knowledge are necessary if PAQs are going to build the community strategies that ultimately improve clinical outcomes. The first challenge to implementing change, PAQ by PAQ, occurs when formerly competing provider organizations try to cooperate for the first time. Focusing on PAQs will break down the individual competition, but community-wide cooperation must also be fostered. As groups who are ready to cooperate with each other are identified, the partnerships help them to redesign their own operations based on the success of other PAQs. As they organize around disease management, the partnership attempts to ensure each PAQ's success as the physicians bring a new opportunity to the community.

## The Changing Community

Community organizations, particularly hospitals, have also been accustomed to fierce competition. This has been a significant impediment to community-wide cooperation. Without the common interest of the new partnerships, these organizations will be unable to learn the delicate balance between healthy competition and collaboration. In the process of community building, a difficult discovery often occurs. Many partnerships find that communities are not composed of organizations and individuals with similar expertise or even similar values. This problem can be resolved by the partnership if the organizations can be united under a truly common vision. Even disparate or competing organizations who start with the vision that there is a better way to improve the health of the community find it possible to define common benefits for all of the community organizations. As the partnership works to bring a vision before the group, a significant paradigm shift occurs within each organization that shares the vision. New abilities and expectations emerge from successful simple projects. The community partners use the early successes to guide more people toward the common vision. When the community works within an efficient system toward a common goal, tremendous energy is released. Building healthy communities represents the nucleus of change that is the ultimate goal of everyone involved in the new practice of medicine.

### Partners for a Healthy Community

A great example of community energy occurred in rural Anderson County in South Carolina. Multiple community organizations joined together to form "Partners for a Healthy Community." Included on the steering committee for the project was Dr. Jay Buehler, director of the family practice residency program. After a comprehensive assessment of community health risks, health behavior, and perceived needs, a plan for community health improvement was formed. Several projects incorporated the need for physicians to change their established practice paradigms. To increase access to physicians, medical residents reinstated house calls to the patient's home. These family practice residents were assigned to visit the homes armed with a clinic on wheels called the *community health van*. This new approach allowed the physician to determine environmental, social, emotional, and economic issues, which influence potential interventions. After visiting with patients and determining what needs fell outside of their immediate expertise, the physicians had the ability to access an extensive system of volunteers. These committed volunteers of the community worked in partnership with the new practice by providing support in areas less comfortable for the physician. A parish nurse program was added to the health care partnership. While the hospital and physicians remained focused on the components of the formal delivery system, it was the relationship that patients formed with the informal delivery system, composed of parish nurses, community volunteers, businesses, and other community organizations, that brought about increasingly positive outcomes.

The Westside Center was established as an effort to bring positive energy into this geographical area, which was identified to have the poorest health status and most constrained access to health care in the region. The facility that would serve as the center was developed in a newly renovated school, where violence had been common only a few years earlier. The principal had actually been murdered on the front steps, so the school had been closed. In the interim what remained had been vandalized and was unfit for any type of services. The Westside Center now includes various community resources, which assist physicians in the total health improvement of patients. Many of the users of this center remained at risk for very poor health; their access to the health system was usually through overuse of the emergency room. The center began to change this trend by including a community clinic, community policing station, child day care, adult day care, and extensive recreational opportunities.

Through an assessment process, the Partners for a Healthy Community team determined that the risk for depression in the county was significant. This finding explained many behaviors that influenced the patients' approach to seeking medical care. It also explained potential complicating factors relating to disease progression and failed health improvement. Through education, physicians have since become increasingly aware and sensitive to these issues. The patients with a high risk for poor recovery from illnesses due to depression were also assisted to achieve appropriate utilization of services that included public services to achieve cost-effective access and appropriate service delivery. Several projects were planned and several more are under way to extend this concept to adjacent communities. As a result of this collaborative process and the physician partnerships in Anderson County, the community has benefited significantly. The overall health status continues to be tracked and is expected to continue to improve.

## The Health Risk–Driven Approach

The new practice of medicine defines a proactive health risk–driven approach that is different from the event-driven patient care approach of old. As Ivan Illich stated, we must develop "healthy people who live in healthy homes on a healthy diet; in an environment equally fit for birth, growth, healing, and dying" (Illich, 1983, p. 192) This outcry for community development can only be met if enhanced by the full participation of the physicians within the new practice of medicine. The physicians are essential in the clinical management side of the partnership that achieves the improvement of a specific health issue.

This risk-driven approach to health improvement either reduces the likelihood of illness or intervenes in the trajectory of the illness through early detection and treatment. The approach requires that the community adopt a community health risk measurement. If the community has established a collaborative community health council or steering committee, the council's role is often to facilitate the measurement of health risks and develop a prioritized approach to intervention. This initial step typically requires six to nine months. First, the steering committee needs to get organized and begin to find a direction to achieve a reduction in health risks.

### The "Growing into Life" Task Force

For example, this type of planning was started in Aiken, South Carolina, because a staggering infant mortality rate had surfaced within a high-risk population. The effort to change this risk led to the formation of the "Growing into Life" task force. A group of citizens committed to lowering the infant mortality rate and improving the health status of underserved, expectant mothers was assembled. The steering committee directed the efforts of multiple organizations. A complete revamping of the staff training for the health department was accomplished to address prenatal issues. A strong partnership with the police department was also established to encourage expectant mothers in trouble with the law to appear at prenatal check-ups. This combined effort enabled the community to reduce the infant mortality rate by 40 percent. This incredible achievement was the result of risk reduction applied by a strong community partnership with providers, driven by collaboration and information sharing.

The development of these community collaboratives can include physicians from any discipline needed for a specific focus in disease management. In the past, the goal of implementing community-wide disease state management to keep patients well did not seem possible to most physicians. Now, physicians can accomplish reduction of unnecessary health care by using the types of information links and support that only the community can provide. Since the creation of health is often dependent on factors external to the health care system—such as crime, education, housing, and emotional well-being—it only makes sense to take advantage of the community support being offered in these areas.

For example, if a physician treats a patient for diabetes, only to send him back to a home with little or no social support, the critical element of dietary compliance won't be achieved. Or if a severe asthma patient it sent back to a home filled with cigarette smoke and pet dander, the positive outcomes and savings will not be achieved. Or if a community has developed a culture of high fat intake and low exercise, the physician cannot single-handedly inspire change in an individual patient who needs to exercise more. If a community assumes the physician can "undo" any negative impact on health through treatment and medication alone, patients are unlikely to work to prevent their own illness.

Without the community partnership, the physician may still feel pressured to practice medicine in a manner that meets old expectations. Even though the grateful patient rewards the behavior, it only serves to continue the dependency. It is only through the development of a unified vision for health and subsequent community action that physicians can break this cycle. Physicians in the partnership are beginning to see that the positive outcomes in the patients they treat are in part due to community support. The community is also beginning to realize the value of the physician's data to track and encourage healthy behaviors. This partnership keeps patients healthy and in a state of recovery by harnessing previously untapped community assets.

The physicians within this community model become the architects of health and the facilitators of services to improve well-being. This role requires significant leadership skills in all six of the dimensions of the transformation.

## Finding Leadership

To start and sustain a healthy community effort, leadership is required. The process of working together works like any other reinforcing system loop. Leadership is required to get the work going, and then the work itself builds additional leadership throughout the process. To initiate this loop, leadership skills need to be developed before the partnership process begins. As collaborators find specific opportunities for the physicians to use their new leadership skills, the physician leaders' growth is reinforced so it can go on to expand the development of even more leadership.

Although most physicians have always been praised for their ability to excel in academics, they were not necessarily considered leaders. A unique leadership style is needed to build community collaboratives. Stated simply, leadership within communities is the ability to influence volunteer participation. Leadership is not a political, academic, or business designation. Although community collaboratives are made up entirely of teams of leaders, the designations such as councilman, chief executive officer, or doctor do not necessarily command a following. The new community leader possesses the skills to facilitate collaboration to benefit the community. For example, when a physician brings peer physicians into a community project, the physician leader must usually orient and motivate the peers. If all of the providers in the community effort are uninterested in building a partnership with the community, they may not coordinate or participate in agreed-upon collaborative care. Without a common commitment, gross inefficiencies occur in the overall project. The collaborating physicians who are instrumental leaders in the effort to develop a healthy community must also help peers see that their involvement is helping their practice.

Community collaborators and physician partners must have respect for each other and the ability to influence each other. Community leaders assist the physicians in change efforts through organized feedback and communication. Mutual accountability is the cornerstone of the community partnership. Although prior models of health promotion have included accountability factors, none have included a full systems approach that acknowledges the interaction of the multiple components of the community and the physician's practice. Physicians in the PAQ need to understand, not only that the human body is a system, but also that the individual within the community is part of the partnership's system. The PAQ physicians must learn that the most enduring context for healing is the whole system. Realizing that the creation of health is not merely the result of specific interventions, the physician leaders prove that the benefits to their own patients are enhanced when they support the community agenda.

### Trinity Mother Frances Health System

Trinity Mother Frances Health System (TMFHS) is an integrated system bringing the new practice of medicine to Tyler, Texas. TMFHS has demonstrated the power of physician leadership, cooperation, and giving. One hospital and a group of physicians in this community established a family care center to serve indigent women. Previously, the only care option for this underserved population was an overcrowded public health clinic. Within three years, this accountable group of providers achieved a 73 percent increase in the access to prenatal care for this population and created a 71 percent drop in the number of babies requiring neonatal care. Although TMFHS did not use unit-based cost accounting to calculate cost versus savings, they did document a significant decrease in fetal and neonatal morbidity. They were originally motivated to help the community when the press made the need obvious by publishing a story on the seriously underserved low-income women in the area. The family center added the sophistication of the new medicine principles described here through widespread education of the medical staff and clinic redesign driven by the physicians. By adding new aligned incentives for provider success, TMFHS is providing better care while simultaneously strengthening their partnership with the community. If they can sustain their momentum, competing systems will have to join in to remain competitive. Through their leadership they will help define health care reform for small urban centers inside rural America. Child immunizations in the family center went from 1,280 in 1993 to 7,000 in 1996. The formal connections with the community are beginning to expand and strengthen as this new practice philosophy matures. This exemplary effort earned TMFHS the 1997 Texas Hospital Association's Excellence in Community Service award.

### Gun Safety

Some community interventions have a more indirect effect on health status. For instance, in a large Midwestern community, several accidental shootings involving children occurred. A community survey found that numerous residents kept loaded guns in their homes for protection. A program to put the safety latch in the on-position on all guns was initiated by a community task force in an effort to decrease the number of accidental shootings. The pediatric practices encouraged parents to get involved. Since the introduction of the program, accidental shootings have been reduced by 30 percent. The hospital emergency department also recorded a reduction in gunshot wounds, verifying the economic impact of helping the community resolve this health problem. This is a classic example of a program that not only improved community health, but also reduced costs for the new practice of medicine.

### Memorial Hospital

In South Bend, Indiana, a free HMO for uninsured families was established. The HMO, which costs the sponsoring hospital approximately $1 million a year to operate, was offered as a contribution to the community. The operating cost had to be found in revenues created elsewhere. The HMO provided care to 400 families who otherwise would only have had the ER for their primary care access. The HMO was able to manage the families' care and avoid unnecessary ER costs that were not being paid by this population. Memorial Hospital assembled a panel of physicians who were willing to take on the patients at deeply discounted rates. Though these physicians took on these patients partly as a gesture to the community, it also made sense from a business perspective for the new practice of medicine. As a result of government reforms, changes in work status, and the likelihood of Medicaid and Medicare HMO coverage, this formerly uninsured group is likely to be covered by capitated insurance at some point in the future within the health system. Influencing the behavior of the formerly uninsured has been recognized in this community as a critical set of skills. This strategy to manage the care of the underserved aggressively is important to long-term success of the hospital and local physician practices. Because they will be at financial risk for the care of this population in a few years, they are managing and improving their health status now. This cooperative community health care partnership is another classic example of the new practice of medicine in action.

## Allina

Allina health system in Minneapolis, Minnesota recently launched a community-wide initiative to manage pediatric asthma. Because they insure 1,032,000 people through Medica Health Plan, they knew they could have a significant impact by simply initiating the new practice philosophy within this population. However, Allina also has a longer-term vision to be the recognized innovator in improving the health of the communities they serve. They are formally providing encouragement and education to help community groups, schools, and the public health department. This effort actually helps the other competing health care systems as well as their own.

What Allina has recognized is that changing the clinical practice and proving the benefit of this new approach to purchasers was the only way to get the market to focus on improving clinical care as well as lowering costs. By following the Institute for Healthcare Improvement's (IHI) approach to asthma management, Allina has been able to create small, incremental projects based on this proven DSM success strategy. By implementing their strategy with a PAQ type model, they have been able to forge change throughout their massive organization to have a positive impact on the community at large. Barb Davis, Allina's project manager of care management, summarized their success strategy with the motto, "Small groups of people get things done." By focusing on the continuum of care and small projects, they proved that a patient-centered, population-based approach can be organized across a community of any size (Coberly, 1998, p. 22).

All of these examples of leadership from around the country demonstrate that health care organizations can take on the responsibility to promote health in the community. These new health partnerships demonstrate that building a healthy community makes sense both from a business perspective and a clinical one. The PAQ physicians create the expectation for a proactive assessment and intervention during the primary stages of a patient's ill health. These health partnerships lead a team that can partner with the patient, other physicians, community organizations and the community in general. Through this process, the physicians lead the community to improved health.

## Doing the Work of the Community Collaborative

People are the key element of the development of a collaborative community effort. A core group of volunteers must be organized by the partnership as the first step toward improving health status and reducing health risks of a community. This core group acts as a collaborative organization that is critical to the partnership. They monitor community health issues, facilitate the development of task forces, identify duplication of services, and subsequently coordinate community health improvement. When organized properly, they can both coordinate interdependent organizations and individuals in the community while simultaneously addressing global partnership issues with an eye to reduce previously unseen duplication. In addition to this organizational alignment, they are also a part of the new clinical coordination and continuity that is such a significant part of the new practice of medicine. Together, they direct improvement of health status and disease management by developing community continuums of care. These volunteers partner with multiple practices and organizations to enhance the treatment of an individual diagnosed with a chronic illness by coordinating community resources.

This approach can be further explained by using diabetes mellitus as an example of the tremendous impact that the new practice can achieve once the community partnership is complete. The strategy of this community-wide partnership is to improve the treatment, health status, cost efficiency, and well-being of people with diabetes. The community collaborative focuses community resources on specific issues that have the most significant impact on individuals, families, organizations, payer groups, and the total community. The new health care partnership's medical component of the community collaborative gets started by developing clinical pathways, or roadmaps, to address the issues of disease treatment. These pathways not only improve the efficiency and effectiveness of medical care, they define what needs to be measured. In the past, data did not track patients moving in and out of health plans who accessed services at multiple sites. With a committed community it is possible to achieve a common patient identifier. Through a community network of data it is possible for the new practice to use Internet communication to provide the medical measurements and relay them to a hub similar to the CIMCO described earlier.

### Working Together

Cost effectiveness in the new practice will plateau unless the full efficiency possible through community coordination is utilized. Lower-cost community services, such as those offered by governmental agencies and charitable organizations, are included in the overall care plan. Services outside the clinical dimension, such as psychosocial support, are viewed as health care interventions to further affect the practice's success. The clinical services of involved PAQs are also evaluated through comparative data. When proven to be above average, the data of a single PAQ can be used to demonstrate success to the community. The community takes on support for health outside the health care system by allowing the PAQ to analyze the impact of specific entry points for informal but still effective improvements in the whole care of their patients.

For example, a community may have 5 percent of its population diagnosed with diabetes, accounting for approximately 15 percent of total community's health care costs. Although care is being administered that uses clinical pathways within the medical system, many patients still receive care and advice from sources outside of the pathway. This may be a result of changing jobs, health plans, or care sites. These outside influences have an impact on the success of the medical care pathway. In fact, patients unable to access the pathway for psychosocial reasons often experience increased severity of the illness (Vetter and others, 1996, p. 159).

Within the same community an additional 12 percent of the population are at risk for diabetes. If this population is not included in the community continuum of care pathway, the occurrence of the disease will increase. Most of these people are unaware that they are at risk and that actions can be taken to avoid manifestation of symptoms. It is widely accepted that health promotion and preventive care, made available to this population in particular, will delay or eliminate the onset of diabetes. So, preventive education becomes a focus of the PAQ and the collaborative community effort. Through the community continuum of care, this at-risk population accesses health promotion and preventive services through the lowest cost, community-based organizations that can prove that they help the patients. These types of partnerships represent a "win-win" situation for the PAQs and the community, allowing both to operate efficiently and without duplication for the benefit of the community. Early detection, through community partnerships, is a significant factor in increasing quality of life and reducing costs to the practice and the community.

### Measuring the Impact

Information makes this remarkable partnership possible, and measurement, feedback, and learning sustain the effort. The benefits of developing community collaboratives can be defined by key indicators of success. It is also possible to quantify the percentage of success achieved against clear goals in specific areas of medical care. For example, the partnership will define a number of clinical events as a goal. Each event has key indicators that can be measured as the event is successfully completed. As care is delivered, it is then possible to track real experience to calculate the percentage of success achieved. The reports of success taken from analysis of the key indicators measured include

- Number and percentage of patients receiving collaborative delivery of care

- Variation in use of community-wide standards of care

- Number and percentage of patients using traditional and nontraditional care in specific conditions

- Number and percentage of patients accessing health care services

- Number and percentage of patients using lower-cost care settings

- Number and percentage of cases using case managers throughout the course of care

- Frequency that access points are achieved within the system of care

- Amount and percentage of uniform patient education delivered

- Number and percentage of patients fully satisfied

- Number and percentage of dissatisfied patients

Many of the areas that define success for the community partnership document the use of the full community continuum of care. Although each community effort is unique, the events that must occur to define successful care often include the services that the members of the community themselves would want if they were ever to develop the chronic conditions being managed. Key indicators of success are developed one condition at a time, starting with chronic illnesses and the high-risk conditions that lead to them. Terminal illnesses will undoubtedly take precedence as life expectancy continues to reach higher levels. Conditions that respond to nontraditional care methods are good candidates for these community partnerships, especially if the illness is affected by significant socioeconomic factors. Eventually even catastrophic illnesses affecting only a few individuals will be the target of this type of measurement to evaluate support that includes community outreach.

## Implementing a Continuum of Care

Knowledge and training are instrumental in the process of implementing community-wide support across a continuum of care according to quality improvement principles (described in Chapter Five). Information from a CIMCO or data office holds the community effort together through feedback. By emphasizing the vision of a preferred future for the community, the partnership guides the changing roles of constituent organizations with an implementation plan. This allows the project milestones to be managed and moved forward rapidly rather than falling victim to the traditionally slow, incremental progression experienced by most communities.

Communicating the aligned vision encourages the implementation process. Communication must encompass more than newsletters. Success must be planned, and the planning process must include a commitment to implementation and one-on-one communication. Facilitated group dialogues are also required. Throughout the development of community continuums, a fundamental belief in the importance of communication based on facts begins to occur. New rules, processes, and operations must be constantly reaffirmed, reinforced, and recommitted to the vision. To do so requires an extremely high level of accountability for the observation and reporting of the data.

### Coordination Is Everything

To develop a community continuum of care, informal and formal care plans must be combined for the efficient, effective management of a single condition. Education, psychological support, social support, and even economic aid must be coordinated. The availability of these types of support should guide the selection of projects and the potential sites for implementing specific, community-based continuums of care. This ensures that education will be patient-centered and reflect efficient learning environments with a minimal disruption to patient lives. Each specific project will aid the community partnership's ability to launch additional care pathways. This experience with coordination is a key step to bring additional sites for providing care together formally. Each participant in the partnership must initiate and then sustain the communication that is necessary for them to help the others succeed. Examples of sites that must coordinate their efforts include

- Business and the workplace

- Existing community volunteer efforts

- Emergency rooms

- Fire departments, emergency medical services, law enforcement agencies

- Homes

- Hospitals

- Houses of faith, religious organizations

- Libraries

- Local health departments

- Payers

- Pharmacies

- Physicians' offices or clinics

- Prisons

- Public service organizations

- Retail establishments

- Schools

- Senior centers

- Urgent care centers

- Wellness centers

The coordination of services and professionals across specific community sites directs the design process and assures that community-wide involvement includes even the most minor contributors. Sites are integrated according to their ability to contribute to the care path requirements for the specific condition that has been targeted.

### Outlining the Processes That Need Implementation

Community continuums depend on specific community-based processes where steps of providing care can be outlined and then implemented. These processes include achieving community motivation, public education, screening, and detection, as well as health maintenance and improvement. Equally important are the clinical steps of early diagnosis, integrated medical treatment, patient education, and self-care. Within each step of care, specific implementation goals are developed according to the condition focus.

Returning to the example of diabetes management, to achieve implementation, specific actions in the area of community motivation are needed. Public awareness and education campaigns are effective means of motivating the community. Another challenge is the identification of at-risk community members. Strategies may be needed to motivate community members to volunteer to be screened. Diagnosis protocols from the new practice, treatment and education protocols, and health maintenance parameters need to be formally introduced to the community.

An action plan can be developed from these implementation goals to help the community contribute in a coordinated way. A flow chart can be created for the action plan as with any CPI-based improvement project. The real challenge will be collecting the data. Although multiple community organizations can work collaboratively along the flow of the specific steps needed for process change, they will need to confirm that the steps were carried out properly at some point. For example, several groups might work toward the goal of screening a set percentage of the at-risk community. The data on how many people have been screened and how many have not keeps them on track. If the data show that a high percentage were screened, most volunteers will feel rewarded and motivated to continue.

### Clarifying the Needs of the Patient

There is a linear relationship between the community continuum success and the level of collaboration between the community at large and the medical community. If medical professionals already coordinate care effectively through utilizing community organizations, the partnership's CPI objectives are very likely to be successful.

The chances for success are even greater if the opportunities for aligned incentives are already in place.

Project objectives must be clear and connected to the real needs of patients. Focus groups of patients, professionals, and the community support groups related to the patients with the condition being addressed can help ensure that these project objectives are met. The link between provider and community is based on patient need, and understanding this need is invaluable at the design stage.

### Developing Indicators of Effectiveness

By developing a timeline with specific points of measurement, the partnership can track the effectiveness of the continuum of care. The CPI feasibility model (described in Chapter Five) provides a critical and necessary structure for determining how a rapid organization analysis and response can be achieved. As the community continuum goes in place, the feasibility analysis helps identify specific areas, where these weak areas will be found, and what potential adjustments will need to be made.

Specific data management and plans for education are developed at each stage of the continuum and are focused on data access points within each community organization. This coordination ensures that a common message with an agreed-upon vocabulary can be used across the continuum.

The physicians and other professionals in the partnership play a critical role in the development of this community continuum strategy. Physicians act as advisors on the design of the continuum. They also help define the clinical goals, objectives, and indicators for measuring clinical success. These goals and objectives also measure community-wide success. Physicians' involvement in this process assures that the necessary clinical goals are in place to take the patient efficiently through the continuum of care. This process gives physicians the opportunity to develop relationships with the community that are critical for the future success of their practice.

**Ensuring the Success of the Community
Continuum Through a Team Approach**

Designing the community continuum of care can follow many paths but all approaches should begin with an understanding of the community's constituents. These constituents direct the establishment of teams that are small enough to do the tasks before them but large enough to include the key stakeholders. For example, clinical specialists can make up one team within the collaborative that can form subcommittees (smaller teams) to initiate the developmental steps within the continuum. The entire project is usually under the direction of an integrated health team consisting of the appropriate PAQs (physician teams) in partnership with the community and other organizations.

*Design Team*

One design team subcommittee can be formed that is responsible for the development process. Additional participants are added according to the clinical conditions that are to be addressed. Participation from health system management, medical staff, and condition-specific consumers of health care can also be recruited for this team. The design team is the core group that builds the framework for development and provides information and support to the other teams in the process. Initially, a steering subcommittee can determine the priorities to address. Once the priorities are chosen, the design team goes to work. In addition to the design team, several other teams are established within the collaborative. The clinical team, the community integration team, and the data team are all critical.

*Clinical Team*

The clinical team is composed of health care professionals. The role of this team is to assure that existing treatment protocols are appropriately interfaced with community support. As appropriate new protocols are developed, the clinical team brings the appropriate professionals—such as physicians, nurses, pharmacists, therapists, dietitians, technicians, mental health professionals, social workers, and clinical educators—together. Marketing professionals may also be recruited for future promotion activities. The clinical team usually has the responsibility to integrate clinical pathways, care maps, or protocols into the community continuum. The clinical teams also assess the likely impact that process steps within the continuum of clinical treatments may have. Once they have the proper information, this team makes recommendations to the organizations that will be involved in prevention efforts and health promotion.

*Community Integration and Support Process Team*

This is a critical group to include in the team approach. This team is responsible for objectively assessing community services and the ability that each demonstrates as they incorporate new processes within the continuum. This team evaluates the appropriateness and cost effectiveness of each process step that each organization could take. The team creates a description of each step on a timeline. The timeline will be needed to address issues such as demand management. The team is also responsible for monitoring the implementation of the process steps at the community organization level.

*Data Team*

Establishing the data team is another critical component of the team approach. This group starts collecting relevant data after the initial development and design of the project has been outlined. It is responsible for the collection of indicators on an ongoing basis. This team can operate as a subcommittee of the CIMCO or it can be housed separately by some other competent organization within the community. Regardless of where data are managed, the data and results that define the results must be accessible by all the other teams, as information propels the system. The data team works closely with the other development teams to ensure this continuous stream of information from the many sources that comprise the continuum. This team usually manages the central community repository where all the data needed for the success of specific community initiatives are housed. Again, this is a good role for CIMCO to provide.

## Momentum Is Building

Once all of the teams are operating on a timeline, they only need to complete the steps in a timely and cooperative effort to achieve success. There are many examples of success as this model begins to take root across the country.

### Change in Newport News

For instance, in Newport News, Virginia, the medical community became aware of a community-wide concern over the number of individuals with diabetes. It was also apparent that the population determined to be at-risk was increasing. The cost associated with caring for patients with diabetes was the impetus for Riverside Health System to initiate a project to address this issue. A design team was developed with input from patients, physicians, payers, community members, educators, public sector representatives, religious leaders, and other community leaders. All possible community locations where either formal or informal health care was accessed were included to ensure that all information and treatment for diabetes in the area was uniform. A clinical design team and a data team were also developed. The clinical design team provided clinical expertise regarding pathway design in an attempt to decrease differences among individual practitioners. The data team was responsible for data collection, transfer, analysis, and reporting.

Throughout the research and design phase, numerous groups were asked what significant issues should be included or excluded in the community continuum. The groups that were convened included patients with diabetes and individuals who provide patients with support, such as spouses, children, significant partners, and friends. Clinical professionals, individuals determined to be at risk for development of diabetes, the general public, payers, and other psychosocial professionals were also included in the discussion.

What they discovered was that one of the most significant issues in managing the disease was the need to purchase glucose test strips to facilitate appropriate behavioral change in the patient and ensure proper management of the blood sugars. Further, they found that the strips were not covered by insurance plans in the area, even though the cost of the strips was often beyond the financial capacity of the patients. As a result of the cooperative relationship between individuals and organizations within the community, a united group made up of the involved community organizations as well as the providers approached one of the payers. They used the data they had gathered indicating the potential savings if they provided coverage for the test strips. Because of their clear analysis, this group convinced the insurance company to change their policy. In this case, the payer accepted the cost of the test strips. The payer was not pressured by the hospital or the physicians. The payer changed its policy because of the coordination of the community, their involvement in the research, and because the request came from a community made up of the insurance company's current and potential members. This type of success could happen nationwide as the new practice of medicine matures.

## Taking the Right Path

The development of community continuums follows a quality improvement path. Once this step is in place, the core of the design team needs to be mobilized. The implementation of each of the required teams—clinical, community integration support, and data—can be managed by the design team. The directors of each team make up an operational steering committee. Each team must have a plan for success. The process steps of each team are not static. Inclusion of increasing numbers of professionals, as well as ongoing improvements to the continuum, follow a continuous management process.

The development of a community continuum of care addresses efficiency and effectiveness across a comprehensive group of people already organized into natural support structures. The new continuum takes advantage of the current structure of organizations and formalizes their cooperation and coordination. The goal of the community continuum is to deliver a unified message to the patient and their family to increase compliance, awareness, management of demand, and increased quality of life. The community continuum teams extend the physicians' ability to care for the patients in all of the dimensions of health: physical, emotional, social, educational, economic, environmental, occupational, aesthetic, and spiritual. From the perspective of the new practice of medicine, these teams unite the community by building awareness for specific medical conditions. They also help the PAQs implement needed informal interventions to achieve economic success. Working together, they can thwart the onset of disease and ensure sustained recovery after medical treatment has been administered. Because the communities help the PAQs succeed, the PAQs push for the healthier communities. This level of coordination and cooperation in the new practice of medicine is what will begin to resolve the health care crisis.

This chapter has reviewed the steps necessary to achieve a community capable of improving its own health through a coordinated effort with new health care partnerships, Chapter Fourteen focuses on the curriculums needed to provide education for physicians as well as community leaders.

# 14

# The Curriculum for Change

Chapter Thirteen discussed the potential of a community-wide health care continuum based on partnership with the new practice of medicine. This chapter suggests a major revamping of the physician skills needed to lead the transformation. Learning and teaching new skills are required of physicians who want to succeed in this new era. This chapter will outline a curriculum and a strategy for peer recruitment and education that will integrate the practice's success with a healthy community.

The widespread, comprehensive implementation of the new practice of medicine is dependent on physicians thinking more cooperatively. The new physician leaders must take this message to their peers. The challenge is clear, for the right actions will not come from the old skills. These physician leaders are building a new paradigm, and convincing others to join them one physician at a time. Their success depends on their ability to facilitate new ways of thinking and then documenting that new physician behavior has actually resulted in success. Physicians must formally link educating and implementing new actions with reporting their success. The PAQ is the functional work group, and the members of the PAQ must be shown new ways to create an economic advantage rather than practicing the way they always have. New practice physicians in significant leadership roles are designing their own curriculums to prepare for their responsibilities as teachers and transformative leaders. These physicians realize that medical education, while providing excellent training in scientifically based problem solving, did not prepare them to lead high-performance teams or information-driven health care partnerships.

Although traditional medical education has undergone significant changes in some university centers, the skills for the new practice of medicine described here are usually learned during the practicing years. The skills described in this book, although valuable as a set of principles for medical students, require learning from real practice experience. The marketplace is changing so rapidly that it would be impossible for the academic curriculum to keep pace.

Some medical schools are trying to respond to health care trends by emphasizing generalist training, disease state management, and innovative ambulatory education programs. This type of education provides students with a view into the full continuum of care, rather than simply immersing them in the hospital-stay experience. But the challenge of going beyond the illness treatment paradigm remains even for these innovative academic programs. It is still a rarity for medical students to learn critical skills such as information management, outcomes collection, high-performance teamwork, adult learning, time management, business partnerships, marketing, finance, behavioral modification, clinical process improvement, telemedicine, home health care, managed care, and community integration.

## Learning to Learn

Perhaps the most significant needs within a curriculum for the new practice of medicine are training in cooperative leadership and life-long learning. Physicians preparing for the future must not only master new medical knowledge but must also understand themselves and their changed relationships with other organizations that will determine their future. The clinical and financial impact of other organizations and individuals in the continuum of care present a critical learning experience for physicians. Because of this continuous learning environment, the new curriculum can be delivered in real time and during daily work activities. In fact, that is the only way it can be learned. It must be expansive and ongoing, grounded in facts, and dependent on change. The curriculum needs to address more than medical decision making and memorized pathways. It must assist the new practitioners in learning to learn from change. The new curriculums need to go beyond teaching content to teaching physicians how to learn with and from the people with whom they work. The concept of learning to learn or self-directed learning is the most valuable skill that physicians can develop. At times, medical education has been seen as a destination rather than a process. The curriculum for the new practice is dynamic and requires a mastery of the process of learning itself.

## Ask the Physicians What They Need

The curriculums evolving in each health care partnership are unique and draw on the specific needs of those who provide the care. After surveying physicians' needs and concerns across the country, the VHA, Inc. compiled the following list of the barriers physicians face in the changing health care environment (Prather and others, 1999). Their concerns were

- Being able to keep up with technology
- Gaining access to the data necessary for informed decision making
- Developing practice protocols
- Making affiliations, choosing hospital relationships
- Understanding how business principles apply to capitated medical service
- Understanding the importance of teamwork

- Lacking vision

- Groups of physicians "carving out" subgroups of patients for profit

- Conflicting needs of volume versus personalized, attentive care

- Distrusting colleagues, organizations, and payers

- Understanding how to work with hospitals in mutually beneficial arrangements

- Changing economic distributions of revenue

- Varying individual practices

- Excluding segments of the medical community

- Overemphasizing cost of care

- "Overmanaging" care: removing the "art" from medicine

- Maintaining quality care while surviving and thriving financially

Judging from this list, most physicians lack an understanding of the trends and forces of managed care. They need business skills and a more standard approach to achieving higher quality without giving up too much control. To understand and overcome the growing list of dilemmas, physicians need an ongoing and dynamic curriculum. When asked what the goals of such a curriculum should be, physicians wanted to know the answers to the following questions (Prather and others, 1998):

- How is quality defined, and who defines it?

- How do we write a mission statement?

- How can we use data to change patient expectations and behavior?

- How should we get paid for doing these activities?

- How do we figure out how much time we should spend on this kind of work?

- How do we define success?

- How do we track our own outcomes?

- How can a diverse group reach consensus on income and expense distribution?

- How do we gain access to our data?

- How do we solve the distrust between peers, organizations, and payers?

To answer these questions, physicians need the skills of cooperation, information management, accountability, change management, and trust building. The new practices are tailoring skill building and general awareness training programs to build these competencies. But simply meeting the physicians' perceived need for education is not always enough. In our experience, real sustained physician change after isolated training programs has been disappointing. The new curriculums are moving beyond public training by combining the implementation of change with education and reward. They are also including formal change management to counter the resistance to change that always accompanies a large-scale transformation. A recurrent training model for physicians is needed. It needs to be ongoing, and it needs to draw on all six dimensions (described in Chapters Three through Eight) to maintain enthusiasm. These lessons also need to be supported with a faculty and teaching materials. Courses must be taught locally in a safe environment that interfaces with all other health care professionals, businesses, and the community as a whole. The challenge of education is a significant one, yet it is a requirement for overcoming the resistance to change.

## Replacing Assumptions with Facts

Central to any curriculum is an analysis of the assumptions that per-petuate fear and distrust between major groups of providers. As these assumptions emerge during the teaching process, the physicians must be challenged to obtain the facts that will resolve old prejudices and misunderstandings. For example, a group of practicing physicians from Colorado compiled the following list during one of these educational sessions. These are the facts they felt were central to resolving the dilemma of the competition between primary care and specialty care. Their goal was to eliminate old assumptions and build a united continuum of care based on the principles of the new practice philosophy. Their list included

- Know what specific units of costs my hospital and practice can measure to define the cost of care

- Know what units of care are provided by which provider in key diagnoses where privileges overlap

- Define primary care current procedural terminology (CPT) codes, specialty care CPT codes, and those common to both specialist and primary care physician (PCP)

- Define severity of symptoms and illness for PCP treated versus the whole population

- Define who gets paid more for providing the same units of care

- Quantify the number of complications of PCPs versus specialists in the same care path where privileges overlap between PCP and specialist

- Measure total cost of care in patients using referrals versus those following the new care path

- Measure units of cost and time spent by diagnosis, procedure, and physician, adjusted for severity

- Track frequency of treatment per 1,000 patients by diagnosis

These were the core facts that this group felt they needed to resolve distrust. To move forward, these physicians needed to overcome old assumptions, so answering the questions was an important part of their training. Facilitated dialogue, a common reward system, a commitment to win together, and using information to resolve differences are all a part of the training model in the new practice of medicine.

But the new accountability that comes from seeing these facts is not without some risk. To use this approach effectively, physicians need a plan that will build trust and a commitment to reinforce change efforts with a structure that can carry out the plan. Trust builds throughout the organization as reports of the key indicators and their relationship to cost and quality become the subject of daily conversation. The curriculum must include this reporting step. The partnership must develop access to the information and then communicate the answers to the physicians' concerns. This approach includes a communication plan for each organization participating in the creation of the new medicine. To make communication a formal part of education, it is important to develop clear rules to guide the use of this type of data.

## Building a Peer Group of Learners

Prior to starting education that addresses the old assumptions, physicians need to decide with whom they want to study. The early leaders need to recruit motivated peers who will teach each other as well as learn the competencies laid out in earlier chapters. A leadership model developed by Mark David, the CEO of a leadership training company in San Mateo, California that carries his name, provides a good example of the principles behind motivated change (David, 1999). In one of his programs, Coach Approach: Building High-Performance Teams, leadership strategies are seen to depend on the development of group trust. This philosophy, combined with the MRM high-performance principles (Chapter Six), can be used as a guide for building new learning teams of providers and recruiting the right peers.

To create the leadership needed to sustain the new practice, a core group of physicians needs to commit to the change process. That takes trust. The core groups that join together and attempt to build and sustain meaningful actions need more than new skills—they need confidence in each other. Once this core group of physicians understands and commits to the new practice model, they are ready to begin the work of leading their peers to join the effort. The challenge for these enlightened leaders is to recruit a critical mass of colleagues who can share the new practice vision in functional relationships. This PAQ-building strategy is done through positive recruitment instead of exclusion. The acronym TRUST emphasizes the value and focus of the work.

The T in TRUST, Truth, is an elusive concept that is held up as a guiding principle. New medical, ethical dilemmas are a focus for much of the training needed for the new practice of medicine. Because of the dilemmas the practices face, physicians are forced into constant change and must have a clear understanding that they are heading in the right direction, even when things appear to go wrong. Complete honesty and integrity must be embedded in the curriculum design as an organizational standard.

The R in TRUST, Results, is important because success or failure is decided by results. Actions lead to results, and results must be measured, reported, discussed, and sometimes changed. The communication of results is guided by systems thinking. The new practice measures the clinical and financial indicators described in earlier chapters and learns from them to create new and better results.

The U in TRUST, Understanding, along with action, is the key to overcoming inertia. Physicians attempting the new practice need to find the courage to change and to lead others to change. If enough facts and assumptions can be clarified to find understanding and a common ground, actions can be taken, even though all the details may not be available for each decision. Because the challenges have become so complex and the system has become so large, it is difficult to obtain all the details. At some point, physicians must make a decision with the information available. A common understanding of purpose can be more important to progress than the smallest details.

The S in TRUST, Security, is not only needed to risk change, but also is necessary for physicians to be confident in the specific decisions they have made. To find this security, leaders must advance through a qualifying process to identify the specific physician's readiness for change. A major focus of achieving TRUST is helping new physician leaders assess the probability that their peers are secure in the decision to change behavior. And those physicians who can change their behavior to join the new practice of medicine must be found. They need to be recruited as physician leaders, educated, empowered, and rewarded.

The first step is the development of peer assessment skills. This leadership skill is almost as critical as the data that guide the decision-making process of the new practice of medicine. Through this recruitment and training process, physicians decide who will be on the new practice team based on who can cooperate, learn, and then change. Because everyone who is successfully recruited and trained contributes to the security of the practice, the security of each individual also grows. The PAQ structure in Chapter Eleven is a good example of this model.

The final T in TRUST, Today, emphasizes the urgency of the situation. The new practice of medicine will succeed only because of the steps each physician takes today. It is discouraging to observe physicians who are unable to change today as the partnership offers everyone the opportunity to grow. The reality is that all physicians will not find the trust they need to change. The curriculum for change is constantly evaluated by those who can act today. They ask, "What has been done today, how much of what was planned actually got done today, and what has been planned for tomorrow?" Change will remain difficult because physicians are more comfortable doing what is familiar. Their focus is on a patient's care, not on what they should do to succeed in their own careers today. Education must teach these physicians that constantly adjusting to rapidly changing business pressures and doing what is best for the patient day by day go hand in hand.

The focus of education that is capable of building trust requires physicians to find balance. The curriculum must also be integrated into daily practice to be effective. The model of learning that can support those with the courage to lead must always make practical sense. The principles that lead to trust give leaders the structure to teach each other. The goal of training has to help physicians create a group that can recruit others to use the competencies from all six dimensions. Learning and teaching these new competencies to each other creates genuine trust among the peers in the new practice of medicine. Regardless of where the physician is in the evolution toward the new practice of medicine, self-management, business planning, action tracking, trend analysis, recruiting strategies, partnership planning, and follow-up are all survival skills. If physicians are willing to master these skills, they will begin to create the new practice of medicine. If they can be recruited using this approach and then educated, they will not only succeed but will also strengthen the most important professional principle, *integrity*.

## Getting Started

To implement the curriculum for change successfully, professionals who want to gain new skills must cooperate. The strategies for measuring cooperation vary based on the size of the group and the group's goals, but tracking cooperation should be part of the curriculum. The rules of systems thinking and cause-and-effect analysis also apply to planning education. This ensures that cooperation in one part of the system is not creating sacrifice or unhealthy competition in other parts of the system. For example, a focus on one specialty or PCP group might create resistance in competing groups of physicians. The overall system's success, however, is dependent on the creation of many small accountable groups. Groups can be formed from solo practitioners or from subdividing larger groups who joined together to establish contracts for increased market share. The challenge for the partnership is integrating accountable work groups that will build, sustain, and coordinate the strategic advantage of the larger group. There will be a continual redesigning of goals to represent new physician groups as they are added to the overall partnership. Those with incompatible goals will select out.

### Self-Management

The next set of skills in the curriculum for change is in the area of personal high performance and influence over peers. This is what many call *leadership*. This type of leadership requires a commitment to doing what physicians feel is right, coupled with awareness that various business pressures could be driving some peers in another direction. The core group of physicians must first form a clear idea of what they really want to achieve and how many physicians are needed for all of them to succeed. Then they need to decide how they will help specific physicians feel secure in their decision to change by joining the partnership effort. In other words, they need a method to prospect for the right physicians, help them stay aligned with the partnership vision, and expand their potential for success through networking with other compatible physicians. To achieve this step, physicians need data. They must make forecasts at the operational level, assessments about how secure people are feeling, and formal communication plans to spread a common message throughout the partnership.

The success of the new partnerships starts with the individual. The core group should have the skills to identify cooperative behavior in others, convince peers to join the effort, and acquire new practice knowledge. These skills reinforce each other like the three sides of a triangle. If any one of these personal skill areas is absent, the triangle collapses (see Figure 14.1).

### Awareness of Behavioral Style

New habits of behavior can be studied and practiced until they are automatic (as was discussed under the fourth dimension in Chapter Six). The central challenge is to replace controlling, demanding, and blaming behavior with listening, collaborating, and constructive critiquing. Physicians can be taught to listen to and watch the behavioral actions of peers as a way of understanding what personal changes are required to feel secure in working with less than cooperative colleagues.

### Convincing Influence

The ability to influence peers to take a cooperative stance stems from the personal actions of each physician. The core group guides

**Figure 14.1. The TRUST Triangle.**

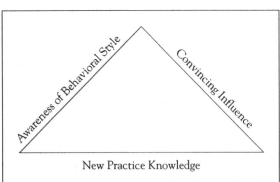

the physician group forward with their maturity, active listening, and keen knowledge of marketplace forces.

The competition is probably offering physicians different opportunities, so the new physician leaders should learn what management service organizations (MSOs), physician practice management companies (PPMs), and staff model HMOs are offering their peers. Physician leaders must ask themselves why the new practice partnership is better than these other opportunities, and they must be genuinely convinced by the answer. To convince their peers that their practice offers the best opportunities, physician leaders must first gather the facts that will soundly convince them. It is important for peers to see the factual answers to their concerns in reports that can be discussed on a monthly basis. These facts are often all it takes to convince peers that they are on the right track.

### New Practice Knowledge

New practice knowledge is the foundation for success, and therefore is the base of the triangle. It requires experience in all six of the dimensions to create the knowledge base that is necessary to move the practice toward the best care possible. When the health partnership is ready to add new physician partners, physicians can use their own skills of observation to decide which peers are likely to make positive change. Because leaders are aware of the alternatives their peers are considering, physicians can discuss their options openly and demonstrate that they intend to help each other choose the best option. And by offering their new practice knowledge to help their peers, it rapidly becomes clear who is ready to change. At that point, physicians can then be recruited to the practice with the confidence that they will contribute to the partnership.

It is a mistake to assume that whoever wants to join the partnership is going to make a good partner. Physician leaders need to evaluate whether an individual is a team player, responsive to quality data, and driven by commitment to the new vision. As leaders, the core group of physicians is also accountable for the new responsibility of building and managing the PAQs. Recruiting new physicians to the overall partnership should be based in part on their peers' willingness and ability to prove they can change outcomes as a working group. It is the experience gained in changing the PAQ's outcome that leads to overall success.

Unfortunately, it is much easier to fail than to change, so the recruiting and educational process take patience. Failure can be accomplished by simply staying the same. To succeed in the information era, physicians must continue to support change even if past changes have not worked. With the new practice knowledge, physicians have the confidence to make changes driven by facts and critique based in cooperation and candor with a group of physicians that are capable of supporting each other and maintaining trust.

## The Teaching Plan

This high level of confidence needed to achieve the new practice dictates the construction of a plan to teach. Writing down a plan and working to implement it will bring stability to the process of leading others. For example, educational content packaged into teachable units over a timeline should include information on the location, faculty, objectives, measures of success, and outlines for workshops, retreats, grand rounds, and speaking events. The partnership demonstrates its ability to succeed through the actions taken by its members, so focusing on the partnership's actions is always part of the teaching plan. Openness, honesty, and integrity are central to this type of feedback if building trust is to be achieved. If physicians do not believe the actions of the new practice are personally achievable, they will not trust the partnership and they will not choose to join the new practice.

A critical discipline that physicians must learn is to find solutions to the problems facing individual practices. The physician's ability learn to create a plan for change and then achieve it marks the turning point for each individual practice. This kind of problem solving carried to completion is tracked as an indicator of success during the education. The teaching plans include a method for solving the problems discovered, creating new approaches, and then implementing new strategies. The milestones that mark success are managed over a timeline.

All too often, physicians neglect to take the time to plan education properly. They may forget that this step is required to be able to measure what the practice achieves after education goes into place. To evaluate the partnership's success, the designers of education must take into account financial forecasts, satisfaction surveys, and the key clinical indicators that outsiders are using to evaluate the practice. By using educational experiments and measuring change in these indicators, a dynamic redesign of the curriculum becomes possible.

The advice contained in this book can be used as the curriculum content guide within the six dimensions of the new practice. By asking what skills and structures are needed at each of these levels, a specific teaching plan can be created. The details on how to put the steps in place to achieve each dimension and how to use the new tools wisely will be unique to each partnership.

### Building Confidence in Peers

To teach within the new medicine, leaders must go beyond technical knowledge and help their peers learn to cooperate, listen, and learn from each other. A physician leader must help peers find the courage to change despite significant outside constraints. The rapidly changing environment makes it difficult for physicians to analyze options and determine direction. It will be confusing and difficult to implement change at the necessary pace. Without feeling confident in their partners, physicians may make decisions that will place their livelihoods at risk.

The physician leaders of the new practice are giving their peers the opportunity to find meaning in their work. The courage to face an uncertain future is not only the result of education but also emerges from strong relationships. Building the necessary courage takes practice, peer support, a new awareness of group behavior, and a concerted effort on the part of the partnership.

## Expanding the Curriculum to Build a Learning Community

A learning community is made up of all of the organizations that are involved in a community health partnership committed to learn from themselves. Peter Senge popularized the concept of learning organizations as he described the five organizational disciplines necessary for continuous learning (Senge, 1990). Each organization within a learning community needs to have the ability to think systematically by using cause-and-effect analysis. They must be committed to teamwork that is focused on a shared vision; in this case, community health. In the ideal circumstance the individuals in these organizations would follow Senge's principles by being committed to achieving personal mastery with truth as a guide; however, these last principles are impossible to measure for an entire community. The participating organizations need to be committed to using shared facts to see the cause-and-effect principles that affect their own success as well as the health of the community. As a learning community the organizations must be able to figure out how they can learn from each other.

Retreats and educational workshops are needed to share, plan, and strategize within the learning community. Learning in the new community is always enhanced with personal experience, rather than by simply asking individuals to memorize new roles. Even as one curriculum is developed, published, and implemented, the partnership realizes that the environment the curriculum was based on has already changed. Physicians should be encouraged to develop specific leadership skills in tandem with skills in self-directed learning. This more global approach to learning allows flexibility and helps the partnership sustain a systems approach to learning and change.

To build a broad learning community that complements the new practice of medicine, partnerships follow the same guiding principles of educational planning used by the PAQs. Information based on reliable data replaces assumptions, as cause-and-effect systems of thought make accurate forecasts and predictions. With systems thinking, the learning community organizes the most effective way to communicate until the curriculum helps the system become a sum of the system parts. A unified learning community for health not only benefits individuals through improved health status but also benefits individual organizations, medical practices, and sub-communities within the larger community. The development of a learning community for health allows the physicians to determine their own destiny and involve themselves in the community's shared vision of the future.

### Community Collaboration Through Education

Successful physician groups will master the skills needed to develop community collaboration and cooperation through workshops and retreats. First, physicians must outline why the improvement of health status can only be accomplished within a system. It should be clear that the separate parts do not need to lose their individuality and identity. Teaching an appreciation for diversity is a part of the grand vision.

For example, to teach interdependence one large group practice conducted a retreat to build community awareness and identify likely community collaborators. The physicians decided that they wanted to be the health improvement leaders. Rather than waiting for the hospital or health department to initiate the process, they realized that being proactive would not only be helpful to their practice but also to them personally. With off-the-shelf computer software, the group analyzed data, information, and perceptions regarding the critical community health connections currently in place. Gaps in community health care were identified, and the physicians could see the important coordination challenges that their diverse community offered. The next step was to bring all the key stakeholders together to help them evaluate their commitment to changing community health. With stakeholders like public health, home health, nursing homes, and schools working interdependently, critical connections became visible. At that point, a communication plan was designed to bring together the critical and most cooperative organizations faster and more effectively.

### Accessing and Guiding Community Information

An evolving skill within the new practice partnerships is the ability to understand what information is held in the community. Each day, the members of our communities are producing more of their own data and are gaining access to mind-boggling amounts of information. Mortality and public health data, disease-specific clinical information, comparative length of stay outcomes data, credentials verification, critical pathway results, peer review data, patient profiles, medical procedure rates, statistical analysis of community interventions, and other community health data are all going on-line through the Internet. The same onslaught of information once only available to the physician is now readily available to community members as well. Data are so widely available that many physicians and much of the community are giving critical consideration to confidentiality issues. In some cases the fear has pushed people to begin hiding data, with good reason. To be actively engaged in the learning community for health, the partnership must recognize the limitation in their ability to educate the public as to the proper use of these data. Community partnerships will need, instead, to develop communication channels that can guide the community and counter the public's misperceptions. It will also be important to focus on getting data from hidden resources in the community, such as data on absenteeism and productivity in the workplace. Links between organizations will also be critical to ensure clarity within the chaos of too much data. These skills are most effectively taught one-on-one with specific examples that show why using the right data in the right way is so critical to achieving the vision of improving community health in the future.

### Building a Structure for Greater Community Impact

Currently many organizations are in the midst of what they call *reengineering* a healthy community agenda. (Although this assumes that these organizations were purposefully engineered in the first place!) Development of a new structure for change, in the midst of too much information input, will require purposeful engineering of a communication structure based on the needs and perceptions of system components. For example, physicians, hospitals, and health systems in the past accessed data from the outside to improve internal process and structure. In the best of circumstances, this evaluation occurred every three to five years. In the new practice of medicine, the health system will be continuously accessing key information internally to see how it affects the whole community. Many data structures within the hospital and physician's office will be linked to the community through a growing network of Internet and Intranet hook-ups. Each learning community for health will create its own unique structures and networks that will be redesigned based on the opportunity found in each of the communities.

Several core components, however, are critical. First, the partnership must view the community as housing the actual health improvement organizations, instead of believing that the health care system is nonexistent in the community. People within the community system will continue to experience ill health, but the focus of improved health within the global system will be based on a structure that can create a summary of clinical data. With this in mind, the physicians are expanding their sphere of influence to shape the data selection as they adopt this larger vision. To be fully effective in a community, extension components of medical care that are currently on the inside of the hospital and physician's office are going to move out into the community.

## Teaching Volunteers

The use of volunteers outside the hospital is an example of how diverse the curriculum for change will become. The volunteer workforce of any hospital system has long been critical to efficient and cost-effective service operations. In the new practice of medicine, volunteers for community health will be educated in the neighborhoods where they live to make a similar contribution. For example, one community in South Carolina has developed Community Health Champions. These volunteers work in their neighborhoods and provide the critical link among the individual, the home, and the rest of the system. Community health champions deliver important information about improving health and quality of life. They help community members access information and services. With this link, physicians can reach individuals before symptoms advance. Costly interventions are held in check, and the chance of negative outcomes is reduced.

In Chesapeake, Virginia, community volunteers are called neighborhood helpers. They have been trained in first-aid and CPR and provide a tremendous service for the community and the new practice. These designated neighborhood volunteer health assistants can be called on in emergencies, but are mostly trained for performing health promotion activities such as blood pressure checks, cholesterol screening, and safety education.

Community volunteers and physicians provide the most basic structure for building a learning community for health. Other health professionals are also important, but the greatest impact will come from volunteer efforts extending physicians' skills. Volunteers are most effective when developed into networks that can communicate what support is needed and provide informal educational efforts. These volunteer networks will teach and coordinate community volunteers, schools, and programs within the religious community and government.

### Community Health Research

Care competencies of cooperative clinical medicine, information management, and the business aspects of the new medicine will be taught in the community in this far-reaching curriculum. The physician will probably ensure that community health research is ongoing. These physicians' efforts will be linked closely with information system skills and community health training. Those physicians with the ability to analyze cause-and-effect clinical relationships via applicable statistical analysis within the community will ensure their leadership roles. Many of the community examples cited in Chapter Thirteen offer specific research opportunities to the community.

### Quality Improvement

Critical performance improvement skills can be added to most learning activities, whether they are limited to specific procedure or process, or expanded to the whole community. Building a learning community for health can be structured as an enormous performance improvement project. The principles needed to organize this effort can be drawn from Chapter Five. The specifics of CPI feasibility analysis are simply conducted in broader and more interconnected projects.

## Finding Noneconomic Incentives

A curriculum for change should ultimately be focused on efforts to develop nonmonetary incentive systems because the future undoubtedly will hold financial constraints. As resources are compressed within the current market, it will become increasingly difficult to provide monetary compensation for the development of leadership skills and their successful application to savings within the community. The strategy for aligned incentives will get the partnerships started, but soon other incentives will be required. The partners will need to determine what incentives should be implemented in each community.

One might consider what factors motivate physicians to participate in training and educational activities beyond the dollar. It may be to improve satisfaction within their practices, improve their personal quality of life, or see visible proof that their efforts have improved the community's health. The next question to consider is, "What does the community need from physicians?" The community of an insured population, the geographical community, and even a community of allied health care providers all need the security that physicians will be available when they are needed. Because access and services are no longer guaranteed, the community's primary incentive to help the new partnerships may become ensuring that the care will be available.

Perhaps special legal considerations will be bestowed upon practices that can prove their success according to the new partnership principles. The success of the new medicine depends on the ability of physicians to lead the development of a learning community for the purpose of health. This success at the partnership level with measurable and public outcome criteria could make accountability less problematic.

The skills described in this chapter are more easily learned and developed in concert with each other under an integrated curriculum. Within a modular approach to learning, all interdependently linked groups can learn and practice new skills with a common focus of achieving the same outcomes and goals. Perhaps collegiality itself will be enough of a reward to sustain the partnerships.

Although self-interest and a failure to understand the interconnectedness of all the key players in the community might weaken and sidetrack the learners within this curriculum, the education process has already begun. The opportunity for physicians to lead this effort coupled with incentives to do so immediately will advance public health in ways never thought possible. But sustaining the new commitment to health as reimbursements continue to decline will be the greatest ethical challenge that medicine has ever faced.

As access to information grows, the public will view "winning" practices as those with motivated physicians that partner to improve community health. These practices will consist of providers who have preserved their profession in service to their community. That may be enough for these physicians to sustain the gains.

This chapter has described the tremendous need for an organized and comprehensive reeducation of medical providers. Chapter Fifteen concludes the book with a quick overview of the transformation of medicine and a final look at the personal challenges that all physicians face as they contemplate their future.

# 15

# A Concluding Message

The six dimensions critical to the next generation of medical care delivery cannot be separated from the public's expectations. The new speed, accuracy, and accessibility of information as supported by the Internet is creating an overwhelming hunger for knowledge. The public has learned that medicine and physicians are imperfect, and the national regulatory bodies have decided that the public has a right to compare the outcomes data of providers. Patients have been given a "bill of rights" by the American Medical Association and others that will include freedom of choice after patients have reviewed the data. Therefore, providers must review their own data and improve outcomes prior to public comparisons. But the economic strategy that would incentivize physicians to do their own measurement has been too far removed from the day-to-day practice of medicine for most physicians to get involved. Practices must be linked together with a clear, economically based reporting system. Fortunately, with the new technology it is possible to organize, sort, and report the overwhelming mass of data into user-friendly interactive messages that can drive improvements with facts and aligned incentives.

This new opportunity can only be fulfilled by creating the right partnerships and basing them on trust. In the new era physicians will be responsible for creating the current drastic state of affairs or the solution. Using systems thinking to predict results before they occur gives physicians the chance to overcome the distrust and confusion that has been perpetuated through faulty assumptions.

By learning from successful practices that are already reshaping their future through incentivized improvements, physicians who grieved the loss of autonomy and control are discovering new enthusiasm. These new partnerships are based on the ethical premise that they will do no harm as they demonstrate visible fairness to each other. By gathering data cooperatively and sharing it systematically, the total, systemwide impact is being calculated. When the data show the need for change, the smallest accountable partnership, the PAQ, becomes the focus for immediate change. Because this approach is bottom-up and linked by the communication of economically critical clinical improvement data, the PAQ can respond to the information with immediate action. The old top-down model of leading big organizations will never work in today's health care environment. The challenge for this generation of physicians is collaborating under a cooperative, data-driven strategy.

CPI is simply the best method for bringing clarity and accuracy to the observation of medical care in real practice. By focusing data collection on clinical decisions, economics, and results, it is possible to stand behind the ethical dictum, "We will do no harm." Even though providers will never be perfect, mistakes can be systematically remedied in the confidentiality of the PAQ as they are exposed. This balance of confidentiality, rapid access to results, and effective means of improving prior to the public comparisons of providers, gives PAQ physicians the leverage to stay on top. The PAQ's success is only possible because these interdependent physician thinkers are rewarded for cooperation after reviewing reliable data and information. Reports on the bottom line verify financial reality and comparisons of disease state management clarify best practices that are emerging within the partnership. This commitment to using facts to help small groups of providers build trust sustains the long-term relationships that are needed for overall success of the new partnerships.

Formal efforts to replace controlling behavior with cooperative, high performance are prompted by fact-based decisions and financial forecasts that create successful business partnerships. The clinical and cost data are organized into reports that help to facilitate timely, accurate communications. Because accountability forces organizations to deal with previously hidden problems, a strategy to support new solutions must be put in place.

A policing or punitive approach to force accountability and improvement always creates resentment and resistance to change. Creating a culture dedicated to cooperative sharing of confidential, individual data builds trust if, but only if, physicians feel safe enough to confront differences of opinion. Partnerships must replace opinion and assumptions with facts and information that reward change in an environment where differences are resolved rather than ignored. By assisting those who have the most room to improve, through careful communication from those who have improved the most, everyone wins. Because rewards are given to a partnered group rather than individuals, comradery and helpfulness without malice are possible. The skills of critiquing, cooperative decision making, and resolving conflicts are taught to small accountable units. Once these skills have been adopted by the PAQ the evolution toward home health and family-centered care is a natural result of the cooperative strategies.

The power of the transformation results from the individual's ability to learn from data, improve outcomes, and then prove that the current outcomes are better than those that were considered the norm. This model is an alternative to rationing and wrongdoing. This learning process will sustain the new medicine when human error inevitably results in isolated blame.

## The Solution

But strategy does not provide the entire solution. The partnership must also put the proper structure in place.

## The Right Partners

Physicians can ensure their future if they can create the right partnerships. There are some very basic principles to follow to find these partners. Trust is needed, and it is far easier to build trust than to find it after it has been lost. A simple rule is to ask the question, "Who or what group can you share information with so that they will share information with you, and create the opportunity for both of you to give more to the community you serve?" This practical definition of true partners will bring people together who can create the integrity needed for the new practice of medicine. Together these giving partnerships can stay focused on mutual benefits and visible fairness.

## Cause and Effect

Partners must also realize that all actions create reactions, and that nothing is truly coincidental. As each partner begins to use systems thinking to discuss the impact of change, new perspectives will emerge and conflict will be inevitable. Because of varying circumstances facing the different partners, there will be many dilemmas that do not have clear solutions. Partnerships that believe in their vision and constantly seek fairness will find it helpful to focus on cause-and-effect processes rather than judging themselves on constantly changing expectations. With access to one another's confidential data, trusting partners are able to find improvements rapidly that others without the same data cannot.

The partnership must be committed to finding win-win solutions to the dilemmas that they face. If the intention is to share data, build trust, and use cause-and-effect relationships to define best practice and economic fairness, then that intention should be held up for all to see. The clear and measurable success factors that are the partnership's goals provide a guiding intention. By finding these common success factors and measuring them regularly and frequently, the progress achieved will reinforce the belief that this dynamic approach to health care reform is the right approach. New goals guide new success, but it is the intention to achieve visible fairness that drives the partnership.

### The Process

The ultimate destination is not as important as the process of getting there, but the process involves overcoming the self-interest and battles that have limited everyone's potential in the past. Staying true to the process of cost and quality improvement, even when the exact partnership outcome is uncertain, will keep the partnership moving in the best possible direction. As the self-interest of all parties merges into the common interest of the community, it is the belief in the process of data-driven positive change that makes the transformation complete.

## Epilogue

The concepts presented here are not theory. All have been proven in some area of this country. However, there are obvious, powerful forces working against this transformation, not the least of which are self-interest and fear. Even the chaotic size of the health care industry will pose a formidable challenge as the transformation overcomes inertia.

As with all paradigm shifts, it will take time for the new rules to be accepted, but with emerging technology the speed of this transformation is likely to be incredibly fast. The physicians who hold on the most tightly to the old rules of physician behavior will probably lose in this health care transformation. Success is available to all physicians, but not everyone will volunteer to change, even to ensure their own survival, let alone success.

This dilemma poses a threat to the transformation process that can best be described through metaphor. The new practice of medicine and the new health care partnerships are like lifeboats. And the old medicine described here is like a sinking ship. Picture a large ocean liner capsized with hundreds of physicians standing on the sinking hull and lifeboats full of medical supplies rapidly floating away from the boat. Each lifeboat will hold thirty or more physicians, but the ocean is rough. In fact, it was the rough weather that capsized the ocean liner and released the lifeboats.

You feel the water and it is cold. You think you may have seen a shark, but you're not sure. In the distance you see land and realize that this was your original destination. The people on land are waiting for your help and the medical supplies you are trained to use. You realize that the drifting lifeboats are unlikely to reach those who need care without your direction. A few of your colleagues have already jumped into the cold water and some are rapidly approaching the security of the lifeboats. You also see one of these brave souls struggling against the current, only to be attacked by the waiting jaws of a shark. You watch as more of your colleagues jump into the dangerous water as the boats drift further and further away. Some are making it to the boats, some are not. To get to the lifeboats, you must swim a long way through shark-infested waters. But you are convinced you can make it. After all, your purpose is to reach land and help the people there. You are about to risk the plunge into the cold ocean when someone from the larger group says, "Wait, the ship can't sink. If we just stand together over on this one side, we can keep it afloat." You notice that many of them are already up to their knees in water, when only minutes ago the hull was dry. You look back to the lifeboats and then down at the ocean.

One of your peers yells, "Traitor!" You glance back and see the angry looks as you move closer to the edge of the hull. The lifeboats have now drifted far enough away that the decision must be made now or never. Three questions haunt you.

"Should I swim as hard as I can to do what I believe is right, accepting the uncertainty and danger? And can I accept the idea of abandoning those peers who will not come with me?"

The last question is the most penetrating of all. "Will I feel better if I stay? At least I will be able to say, 'We went down together.'"

The choices in this metaphor are very similar to those facing physicians. The opportunity for physicians to lead the new practice of medicine will never enjoy a greater likelihood of success than it does today. Yet when there is little pain from managed care the motivation to take risks is not found in many practicing physicians. When the pain of decreasing income and increasing hassles is great enough, the motivation will increase, but the work required to create the new practice of medicine will be much harder. Those who can act from wisdom rather than fear will reach the opportunity they want with strength and courage. Those who wait too long may find that the proactive physicians have already joined together and created the best partnerships. Once the best partnerships are established, they will only expand if their data show it is wise to do so. At that point, the opportunity to be on the winning side might be gone. Those who succeed at this model will miss their colleagues who were unable to change with the times. Once established in the new practice, these successful physicians will remember that their decision was available to those who stayed behind. With information, accountability, ethically driven action, and proof that they are serving the community within an economically successful practice, they will realize that they deserve to succeed. Going back to the old model of medicine will not be an option. They will look back on the past as history but reflect on the benchmark successes that they are creating as they build the future. They will endure, not because they took anyone's place, but because they acted from integrity and found the courage to lead!

# References

## Chapter One

Ackerknecht, E.H. *A Short History of Medicine*. Baltimore, Md.: The Johns Hopkins University Press, 1982.

Burnham, J. C. "American Medicine's Golden Age: What Happened to It?" *Science*, March 19, 1982, 1474–1479.

Diabetes Control and Complications Trial Research Group. "Lifetime Benefits and Costs of Intensive Therapy as Practiced in the Diabetes Control and Complications Trial." *Journal of the American Medical Association*, 1996, *276*, 1409–1415.

Eddy, D. M. "Clinical Decision Making: From Theory to Practice. Rationing Resources While Improving Quality: How to Get More for Less." *Journal of the American Medical Association*, 1994, *272*, 817–824.

Goldsmith, M. F. "National Patient Safety Foundation Studies Systems." *Journal of the American Medical Association*, 1997, *278*(19), 1561.

Halvorson, G. C. *Strong Medicine*. New York: Random House, 1993.

Hannan, E. L., and others. "Improving the Outcomes of Coronary Artery Bypass Surgery in New York State." *Journal of the American Medical Association*, 1994, *271*(10), 761–766.

Perlman S. E. "Judge: MD Ranking Can Go Public." *Newsday*, Oct. 22, 1991.

Scofea, L. A. "The Development and Growth of Employer-Provided Health Insurance." *Monthly Labor Review*, March 1994, 3.

Sidel, V. W., and Sidel, R. *Reforming Medicine: Lessons of the Last Quarter Century*. New York: Pantheon Books, 1984.

Star, P. *The Social Transformation of American Medicine*. New York: Basic Books, 1982.

Williams, S. V., Nash, D. B., and Goldfarb, N. "Differences in Mortality from Coronary Artery Bypass Graft Surgery at Five Teaching Hospitals." *Journal of the American Medical Association*, 1991, 266(6), 810–815.

# Chapter Two

Center for the Evaluative Clinical Sciences, Darmouth Medical School. *The Dartmouth Atlas of Health Care*. Chicago: American Hospital Publishing, 1996.

Classen, D. C., Evans, R. S., Pestotnik, S. L., Horn, S. D., Menlove, R. I., and Burke, J. P. "The Timing of Prophylactic Administration of Antibiotics and the Risk of Surgical Wound Infection." *New England Journal of Medicine*, 1992, 326(5), 281–286.

Classen, D. C., Pestotnik, S. L., Evans, R. S., and Burke, J. P. "Computerized Surveillance of Adverse Drug Events in Hospitalized Patients." *Journal of the American Medical Association*, 1991, 266(20), 2847–2851.

Cohan, C., Pimm, J. B., and Jude, J. R. *A Patient's Guide to Heart Surgery*. New York: Harper Collins, 1991.

Forrester, J. *Industrial Dynamics*. Cambridge, Mass.: MIT Press, 1961.

Goleman, D., and Gurin, J. *Mind/Body Medicine: How to Use Your Mind for Better Health*. Yonkers, N.Y.: Consumers Union of United States, Inc., 1993.

Leape, L. L. "Error in Medicine." *Journal of the American Medical Association*, 1994, 272(23), 1851–1857.

Millenson, M. L. *Demanding Medical Excellence*. Chicago: The University of Chicago Press, 1997, pp. 80–89.

Paich, M. "Generic Structures." In *System Dynamics Review*, Summer, 1985, 1, 126–132.

Pestotnik, S. L., Classen, D. C., Evans, R. S., and Burke, J. P. "Implementing Antibiotic Practice Guidelines Through Computer Assisted Decision Support: Clinical Outcomes and Financial Outcomes." *Annals of Internal Medicine*, 1996, 124(10), 884–890.

Senge, P. M. *The Fifth Discipline*. New York: Doubleday Currency, 1990.

Von Bertalanffy, L. *General Systems Theory*. New York: George Braziller, 1968.

# Chapter Three

Cleveland, W. S. *The Elements of Graphing Data*. Summit, N.J.: Hobart, 1994.

Shortell, S. M., and others. *Remaking Health Care in America: Building Organized Delivery Systems*. San Francisco: Jossey-Bass, 1996.

# Chapter Four

Brennan, T. A., and others. "Incidence of Adverse Events and Negligence in Hospitalized Patients: Results of the Harvard Medical Practice Study I." *New England Journal of Medicine*, 1991, *324*(6), 370–376.

Halvorson, G. C. *Strong Medicine*. New York: Random House, 1989.

Richards, E. P., and others. "Physicians in Managed Care: A Multi-Dimensional Analysis of New Trends in Liability and Business Risk." *Journal of Legal Medicine*, Dec. 18, 1997, 443–473.

Solomon, R. J. *The Physician Manager's Handbook: Essential Business Skills for Succeeding in Health Care*. Gaithersburg, Md.: Aspen, 1997.

# Chapter Five

Berwick, D. (ed.). Review of 1998 Publications. *Eye on Improvement*, Dec. 1998.

Blumenthal, D., and Scheck, A. *Improving Clinical Practice*. San Francisco: Jossey-Bass, 1995.

James, B. C. *Quality Management for Health Care Delivery* (monograph). Chicago: Hospital Research and Educational Trust (American Hospital Association), 1989.

James, B. C., Horn, S. D., and Stephenson, R. A. "Management by Fact: What Is It and How Is It Used?" In S. D. Horn and D. Hopkins (eds.) *Clinical Practice Improvement: A New Technology for Developing Cost Effective Quality Health Care*. New York: Faulkner & Gray, 1994, pp. 39–54.

Morris, A. H., and others. "Randomized Clinical Trial of Pressure Controlled Inverse Ratio Ventilation and Extracorporeal $CO_2$ Removal for Adult Respiratory Distress Syndrome." *American Journal of Respiratory Critical Care Medicine*, 1994, *149*, 295–305.

Prather, S. E. *VHA Physician Leadership Program: Module III, Appendix A*. Irving, Tx.: VHA Inc., 1998.

Siegel, R. H. "Contempo New and Now: Updates Linking Evidence and Experience." *Journal of the American Medical Association*, 1998, *279*(17), 1395–1396.

# Chapter Six

Argyris, C. *Strategy, Change, and Defensive Routines*. Boston, Mass.: Pitman, 1995.

Blake, R. R., and Mouton, J. S. *Corporate Excellence Through Grid Organization Development: A Systems Approach*. Houston, Tx.: Gulf, 1968.

Blake, R. R., and Mouton, J. S. *Grid Cockpit Resource Management*. Austin, Tx.: Scientific Methods, Inc., 1984.

Carothers, N. B. "Medication Errors: The Problem and Its Scope." *International Journal of Trauma Nursing*, Sept. 1998, 104–108.

*The Cockpit*, United Airlines, March/April, 1986.

Csikszentmihalyi, M. *Flow: The Psychology of Optimal Experience*. New York: Harper & Row, 1990.

Gerety, R. "Why Now Is the Time for CPI: A Physician's Perspective." In S. Horn and D. Hopkins (eds.), *Clinical Practice Improvement: A New Technology for Developing Cost-Effective Quality Health Care*. New York: Faulkner & Gray, 1994.

Goldman, S. L. "Assessment of Physician Performance of Cardiopulmonary Resuscitation." *Journal of Family Practice*, Feb. 1985, 173–178.

Knowles, M. S. *The Adult Learner: The Definitive Classic in Adult Education and Human Resource Development*. Houston, Tx.: Gulf, 1998.

Kolb, D. A. *Experimental Learning: Experience as the Source of Learning and Development*. Englewood Cliffs, N.J.: Prentice Hall, 1984.

Lavber, J. K. "Resource Management Training for Flight Deck Crew Members." *Resource Management on the Flight Deck*. National Aeronautics and Space Administration, 1980.

National Transportation Safety Board. *Safety Recommendations A–85–26 and 27*, April 15, 1985, 1–5. Washington, D.C.: National Transportation Safety Board.

Prather, S. E., Blake, R. R., and Mouton, J. S. *Behavioral Types and the Art of Patient Management*. Los Angeles: Practice Management Information, 1990a.

Prather, S. E., Blake, R. R., and Mouton, J. S. *Medical Risk Management*. Oradell, N.J.: Medical Economics Company, Inc., 1990b.

## Chapter Seven

Arpin, K., and others. "Prevalence and Correlates of Family Dysfunction and Poor Adjustment to Chronic Illness in Specialty Clinics." *Journal of Clinical Epidemiology*, 1990, 43(4), 373–383.

Butler, R. N., and others. "Type 2 Diabetes: Patient Education and Home Blood Glucose Monitoring." *Geriatrics*, 1998, 60, 63–64, 67.

Davis, P. T., and Hamill, C. T. "Disease State Management: A Proactive Approach to Better Service." *Today's Home Healthcare Provider*, Nov.–Dec. 1997.

Diabetes Control and Complications Trial Research Group. "Lifetime Benefits and Costs of Intensive Therapy as Practiced in the Diabetes Control and Complications Trial." *Journal of the American Medical Association*, 1996, *276*, 1409–1415.

Dougherty, G., and others. "Home Based Management Can Achieve Intensification Cost-Effectively in Type I Diabetes." *Pediatrics*, Jan. 1999, 122–128.

Eliupoulus, C. "Chronic Care Coaches: Helping People to Help People." *Home Health Nurse*, March 1997, 185–188.

La Puma, J. *Managed Care Ethics: Essays on the Impact of Managed Care on Traditional Medical Ethics*. New York: Haitherleigh, 1998.

McCusker, J. "The Use of Home Care in Terminal Cancer." *American Journal of Preventive Medicine*, March-April, 1985, 42–52.

Paradis, L. F., and others. "Hospice: A Rapidly Growing Health Care Delivery Segment." *Michigan Medicine*, March 1983, 180–182.

Persily, C. A., and others. "A Model of Home Care for High-Risk Child Bearing Families. Women with Diabetes in Pregnancy." *Nursing Clinics of North American*, June 1996, 327–332.

# Chapter Eight

Carlson, L. K. "Creating Healthier Communities, Challenge for the 21st Century." *Medical Interface*, 1994, 62–68.

Close, E. J., and others. "Diabetic Diets and Nutritional Recommendations: What Happens in Real Life?" *Diabetetic Medicine*, March 1992, 181–188.

Collis, M. D. "Behavior Modification Techniques: Their Use in Individual and Community Programs." *International Journal of Health Education*, 1977, *20*, 19–37.

Davis, C., and others. "Benefits to Volunteers in a Community Based Health Promotion and Chronic Illness Self-Management Program for the Elderly." *Journal of Gerontology Nursing*, Oct. 1998, 16–23.

Henry, S. A. "Administrative Integration Through Product and Service Line Structure." In M. Tonges (ed.), *Clinical Integration*. San Francisco: Jossey-Bass, 1998, pp. 62–68.

Robinson, J. C., and Luft, H. S. "The Impact of Hospital Market Structure on Patient Volume Average Length of Stay, and the Cost of Care." *Journal of Health Economics*, 1985, *4*, 333–356.

*Utah's Health: An Annual Review*, Vol. 4. Salt Lake City: University of Utah, Governor Scott M. Matheson Center for Health Care Studies, 1996.

## Chapter Nine

Carpenter, L. M., Swerdlow, A. J., and Fear, N. T. "Mortality of Doctors in Different Specialties: Findings from a Cohort of 20,000 NHS Hospital Consultants." *Occupational and Environmental Medicine*, June 1997, 388–395.

Prather, S., and others. *VHA IMPAQ Survey*. Salt Lake City, UT: Medical Resource Management, 1999.

## Chapter Ten

Gutman, J. (ed.). *1999 Disease Management Directory and Guidebook*. Atlanta: National Health Information, 1999.

McNabb, W. L., and others. "Critical Self-Management Competencies for Children with Asthma." *Journal of Pediatric Psychology*, March 1986, 103–107.

## Chapter Eleven

Amschler, D. H. "Pap Tests Every Three Years: Cost Effective in the Long Run?" *Health Education*, Jan.-Feb. 1983, 42–45.

Argyris, C., and Kaplan, R. S. "Implementing New Knowledge: The Case of Activity Based Cost Accounting." *Horizons*, Sept. 1994, 83–105.

Barnett, A. "Integration Leader Friendly Hills Switches Models—Again." *Hospital Health Network*, Nov. 1994, 66–68.

Boulet, L. P. "Asthma Education: What Has Been Its Impact?" *Canadian Respiratory Journal*, July-Aug. 1998, 91–96.

Cochrane, J. D. (ed.). *The Integrated Healthcare Report*. San Diego, 1994.

Holzman, M. D., Elkins, C. C., Neuzil, D. F., and Williams, L. F. "Expanding the Physicians Care Team: Its Effect on Patient Care, Resident Function, and Education." *Journal of Surgery Research*, June 1994, 636–640.

Lumsdom, K. "Why Doctors Don't Trust You." *Hospital Health Network*, March 1996, 26–28, 30, 32.

Stafford, R. S. "Cesarean Section Use and Source of Payment: An Analysis of California Hospital Discharge Abstracts." *American Journal of Public Health*, March 1990, 313–315.

## Chapter Twelve

Bergthold, L. *Purchasing Power in Health: Business, the State, and Health Care Politics*. New Brunswick, N.J.: Rutgers University Press, 1990.

Califano, J. A. *America's Health Care Revolution: Who Lives? Who Dies? Who Pays?* New York: Random House, 1986.

Charles, S. C., and others. "Predicting Risk for Medical Malpractice Claims Using Quality of Care Characteristics." *Western Journal of Medicine*, Oct. 1992, 433–439.

Christianson, J., and others. "Managed Care in the Twin Cities: What Can We Learn?" *Health Affairs*, Summer 1995, 114–130.

Hannan, E. L. "Adult Open Heart Surgery in New York State: An Analysis of Risk Factors and Hospital Mortality Rates." *Journal of the American Medical Association*, Dec. 5, 1990, 2768–2774.

Leape, L. L. "The Appropriateness of Use of Coronary Artery Bypass Graft Surgery in New York State." *Journal of the American Medical Association*, Feb. 10, 1993, 753–769.

Millenson, M. L. *Demanding Medical Excellence*. Chicago: University of Chicago Press, 1997.

Moses, L. E. and Mosteller, F. "Institutional Differences in Post-Operative Death Rates: Commentary on Some of the Findings of the National Halothane Study." *Journal of the American Medical Association*, 1968, *203*(7), 150–152.

Reinertson, J. "The Point Is Transformation, Not Doing Continuous Improvement." *Joint Commission Journal on Quality Improvement*, *19*(10), 1993, 451.

Schneider, E. C. "Influence of Cardiac-Surgery Performance Reports on Referral Practices and Access to Care." *New England Journal of Medicine*, July 25, 1996, 251–256.

Sessa, E. J. "Information Is Power: The Pennsylvania Experiment." *Journal of Health Care Benefits*, Jan.-Feb. 1992, 44–48.

Siro, C. A., and others. "Evaluating Outcomes in Cardiac Care and Developing Consensus for Action: The Pennsylvania Health Care Cost Containment Council Experiment." *American Journal of Medical Quality*, Spring, 1996, 30–34.

Stanford Center for Health Care Research. "Comparison of Hospitals with Regard to Outcomes of Surgery." *Health Services Research* 1976, *11*(2), 112–127.

Wennberg, J. E. "Understanding Geographic Variations in Health Care Delivery." *New England Journal of Medicine*, Jan. 1999, 52–53.

Wennberg, J. E., and others. "Small Area Variations in Health Care Delivery." *Science*, Dec. 1973, *182*(117), 1102–1108.

## Chapter Thirteen

Coberly, S. *Managed Care, Operations and Performance. Innovations in Organized Systems of Care. Health Care Delivery System Reform.* Washington, D.C.: Washington Business Group on Health, 1998.

Illich, I. *Gender.* New York: Pantheon, 1983.

Vetter, P., and others. "Clinical and Psychosocial Variables in Different Diagnostic Groups: Their Interrelationships and Value as Predictors of Course and Outcome During a 14-Year Follow Up." *Psychopathology,* 1996, *29,* 159–168.

## Chapter Fourteen

David, M. *The Coach Approach: Building High Performance Relationships.* San Mateo, Calif.: Mark David Corporation, 1999. Used with permission.

Prather, S., and others. VHA *Physician Leadership Module III Report.* Salt Lake City, UT: Medical Resource Management, 1998.

Prather, S., and others. VHA *IMPAQ Survey Results.* Salt Lake City, UT: Medical Resource Management, 1999.

Senge, P. *The Fifth Discipline.* New York: Doubleday Currency, 1990.

# Recommended Reading

## General Quality Improvement—The Basics

Angell, M., and Kassirer, J. P. "Quality and the Medical Marketplace—Following Elephants." *New England Journal of Medicine*, 1996, 335(12), 883–885.

Berwick, D. M. "Sounding Board: Continuous Improvement as an Ideal in Health Care." *New England Journal of Medicine*, 1989, 320(1), 53–56.

Berwick, D. M. "Eleven Worthy Aims for Clinical Leadership of Health System Reform." *Journal of the American Medical Association*, 1994, 272, 797–802.

Berwick, D. M., Godfrey, A. B., and Roessner, J. *Curing Health Care: New Strategies for Quality Improvement.* San Francisco: Jossey-Bass, 1990.

Blumenthal, D. "Total Quality Management and Physicians = Clinical Decisions." *Journal of the American Medical Association*, 1993, 269, 2775–2778.

Blumenthal, D. "Quality of Care—What Is It?" *New England Journal of Medicine*, 1996, 335(12), 891–893.

Blumenthal, D. "The Origins of the Quality-of-Care Debate." *New England Journal of Medicine*, 1996, 335(15), 1146–1148.

Blumenthal, D., and Epstein, A. "The Role of Physicians in the Future of Quality Management." *New England Journal of Medicine*, 1996, 335(17), 1328–1331.

Blumenthal, D., and Scheck, A. C. (eds.). *Improving Clinical Practice: Total Quality Management and the Physician.* San Francisco: Jossey-Bass, 1995.

Chassin, M. R. "Improving the Quality of Care." *New England Journal of Medicine*, 1996, 335(14), 1060–1062.

Couch, J. B. (ed.). *Health Care Quality Management for the 21st Century.* Venice, Fla.: American College of Physician Executives, 1991.

Crouch, J. M. "Essential Tools for Quality Managers. Or, What I Wish I Knew Before I Took This Job." *Quality Digest*, 1997, June, 24–30.

Deming, W. E. *Out of the Crisis*. Cambridge: MIT Center for Advanced Engineering Study, 1986.

Gaucher, E. J., and Coffey, R. J. *Total Quality in Healthcare: From Theory to Practice*. San Francisco: Jossey-Bass, 1993.

Horn, S. D., and Hopkins, D. S. P. *Clinical Practice Improvement: A New Technology for Developing Cost-Effective Quality Health Care*. New York: Faulkner & Gray, 1994.

James, B. C. *Quality Management for Health Care Delivery* (monograph). Chicago: Hospital Research and Educational Trust (American Hospital Association), 1989.

James, B. C. "Getting the Best Outcome in the Most Appropriate Way: Continuous Quality Improvement Theory." In *Health Care in the 1990s and Beyond: Focus on Outcomes*. Princeton, N.J.: Excerpta Medica, 1991.

Juran, J. M. *Juran on Planning for Quality*. New York: Free Press, 1988.

Kleeb, T. E. "Teaching Total Quality Management: Developing and Deploying Education Throughout a Healthcare System." *Journal for Healthcare Quality*, 1997, *19*(2), 17–23, 26.

Laffel, G., and Blumenthal, D. "The Cause for Using Industrial Quality Management Science in Health Care Organizations." *Journal of the American Medical Association*, 1989, *262*, 2869–2873.

Langley, C., and others. *The Improvement Guide: A Practical Approach to Enhancing Organizational Performance*. San Francisco: Jossey-Bass, 1996.

Mosser, G. "Clinical Process Improvement: Engage First, Measure Later." *Quality Managment in Health Care*, 1996, *4*(4), 11–20.

Walton, M. *The Deming Management Method*. New York: Dodd, Mead & Company, 1986.

Wehlander, T. "Performance Improvement Through Self-Paced Learning." *Journal for Healthcare Quality*, 1997, *19*(4), 26–28.

# Improving Outcomes

Bates D. W., Cullen, D. J., Laird, N., and others. "Incidence of Adverse Drug Events and Potential Adverse Drug Events: Implications for Prevention." *Journal of the American Medical Association*, 1995, *274*, 29–34.

Bell, R., Krivich, M. J., and Boyd, M. S. "Charting Patient Satisfaction: Tracking the Efforts of Patient Satisfaction Efforts with Control Charts Will Add

Value to Your Business Strategy." *Marketing Health Services*, 1997, *17*(2), 22–29.

Carlson, K. J., Miller, B. A., and Gowler, F. J. Jr. "The Maine Women's Health Study. I. Outcomes of Hysterectomy." *Obstetrics and Gynecology*, 1994, *83*, 556–565.

Cherkin D. C., Deyo, R. A., and Street, J. H. "Predicting Poor Outcomes for Back Pain Seen in Primary Care Using Patients' Own Criteria." *Spine*, 1996, *21*(24), 2900–2907.

Classen, D. C., Evans, R. S., Pestonik, S. L., Horn, S. D., Menlove, R. I., and Burke, J. P. "The Timing of Prophylactic Administration of Antibiotics and the Risk of Surgical-Wound Infection." *New England Journal of Medicine*, 1992, *326*, 281–286.

Classen, D. C., Pestonik, S. L., Evans, R. S., and Burke, J. P. "Computerized Surveillance of Adverse Drug Events in Hospitalized Patients." *Journal of the American Medical Association*, 1991, *266*, 2847–2851 [Erratum, *Journal of the American Medical Association*, 1992, *267*, 1922.]

Crain, E. F., Weiss, K. B., and Fagan, M. J. "Pediatric Asthma Care in US Emergency Departments." *Archives of Pediatrics and Adolescent Medicine* 1995, *149*, 893–901.

Curtis, P., Mintzer, M., and Resnick, J. "The Quality of Cervical Cancer Screening: A Primary Care Prospective." *American Journal of Medical Quality*, 1996, *2*(1), 11–17.

Doan, T., Grammer, L. C., Yarnold, P. R., Greenberger, P. A., and Pattersons, R. "An Intervention Program to Reduce Hospitalization Cost of Asthmatic Patients Requiring Intubation." *Annals of Allergy Asthma and Immunology*, 1996, *76*, 513–518.

Emerman, C. L., and Cydulka, R. K. "Effect of Pulmonary Function Testing on the Management of Acute Asthma." *Archives of Internal Medicine*, 1995, *155*, 2225–2228.

Gaioni, S. J., Korenblat-Hanin, M., Fisher, E. B., and Korenblat, P. "Treatment Outcome in an Outpatient Asthma Center: Retrospective Questionnaire Data." *American Journal of Managed Care*, 1996, *2*(8), 999–1007.

Gibson P. G., Wlodarczyk, J., Hensley, M. J., Murree-Allen, K., Olson, L. G., and Saltos, N. "Using Quality Control Analysis of Peak Expiratory Flow Recordings to Guide Therapy for Asthma." *Annals of Internal Medicine*, 1995, *123*, 488–492.

Greenfield, S., Rogers, W., Mangotich, M., Carney, M. F., and Tarlov, A. R. "Outcomes of Patients with Hypertension and Noninsulin Dependent Diabetes Mellitus Treated by Different Systems and Specialities: Results from the Medical Outcomes Study." *Journal of the American Medical Association*, 1995, *274*, 1436–1444.

"Henry Ford Health System Reduces Costs, Enhances Wound Care Management." *Eye on Improvement*, October 15, 1997.

"Hospital-Owned Clinic Reduces Hospitalization and Improves Quality of Life in Congestive Heart Failure." *Eye on Improvement*, November 15, 1997.

Leape, L. L. "Error in Medicine." *Journal of the American Medical Association*, 1994, *272*, 1851–1857.

Malmivaara A., Hakkinen, U., Aro, T., and others. "The Treatment of Acute Low Back Pain—Bed Rest, Exercises, or Ordinary Activity." *New England Journal of Medicine*, 1995, *332*, 351–355.

Mayo, P. H., Richman, J., and Harris, H. W. "Results of a Program to Reduce Admissions for Adult Asthma." *Annals of Internal Medicine*, 1990, *112*, 864–871.

McKay, M. D., Rowe, M. M., and Frank, M. B. "Disease Chronicity and Quality of Care in Hospital Readmissions." *Journal for Healthcare Quality*, 1997, *19*(2), 33–37.

McMahon, M. J., Luther, E. R., Bowes, W. A., and others. "Comparison of a Trial of Labor with an Elective Second Cesarean Section." *New England Journal of Medicine*, 1996, *335*, 689–696.

Niles, N., Tarbox, G., and Schults, W. "Using Qualitative and Quantitative Patient Satisfaction Data to Improve the Quality of Cardiac Care." *The Joint Commission Journal on Quality Improvement*, 1996, *22*(5), 323.

Reily, P., Pike, A., and Phipps, M. "Learning from Patients: a Discharge Planning Improvement Project." *The Joint Commission Journal on Quality Improvement*, 1996, *22*(5), 149.

Rosenstein, A. H., Swedlow, A., and Simon, T. "Benchmarking Outcomes for Diagnosis and AMI: A Multidisciplinary Hospital Performance Improvement Project." *Best Practices and Benchmarking in Healthcare*, 1997, *2*(2), 71–81.

Rosenthal, G. E., Quinn, L., and Harper, D. I. "Declines in Hospital Mortality Associated with a Regional Initiative to Measure Hospital Performance." *American Journal of Medical Quality*, 1997, *12*(2): 103–112.

Scura, K. W., and Whipple, B. "How to Provide Better Care for Postmenopausal Women." *American Journal of Nursing*, 1997, *97*(4), 36–43.

Selby, J. V. "Variation Among Hospitals in Coronary-Angiography Practices and Outcomes After Myocardial Infarction in a Large Health Maintenance Organization." *New England Journal of Medicine* 1996, *335*, 1918–1919.

Weinstein, A. G., Faust, D. S., McKee, L., and Padman, R., "Outcome of Short-Term Hospitalization for Children with Severe Asthma." *Journal of Clinical Immunology*, July 1992, 90 (1), 66–75 (Bibliography: Figure 5.2).

Yamamoto, L. G. "Radiology Cases in Pediatric Emergency Medicine: Amplifying the Benefits of Performance Improvement by Sharing a Hospital Performance Improvement Program with the World via the Internet." *American Journal of Medical Quality*, 1997, *12*(1), 69–75.

## The Challenges of Measurement and Reporting

"AHCPR and Kaiser Examine Consumers' Use of Quality Information." *Research Activities*, December 1996, *199*(97–107).

Ashton, C. M., Kuykendall, D. H., Johnson, M. L., and others. "A Method of Developing and Weighting Explicit Process of Care Criteria for Quality Assessment." *Medical Care*, 1994, *32*, 755–770.

Barry, M. J., Gowler, F. J. Jr., O'Leary, M. P., Bruskewitz, R. C., Holtgrewe, H. L., and Mebust, W. K. "Measuring Disease-Specific Health Status in Men with Benign Prostatic Hyperplasia." *Medical Care*, 1995, *33*, Suppl:AS145–AS155.

Brennan, T. A., Hebert, L. E., Laird, N. M., and others. "Use of Medical Care in the RAND Health Insurance Experiment: Diagnosis- and Service-Specific Analyses in a Randomized Controlled Trial." *Medical Care*, 1986, *265*, 3265–3269.

Brook, R. H., Davies-Avery, A., Greenfield, S., and others. "Assessing the Quality of Medical Care Using Outcome Measures: An Overview of the Method." *Medical Care*, 1977, *15*, Suppl.

Brook, R. H., Mcglynn, E. A., and Cleary, P. D. "Measuring Quality of Care." *New England Journal of Medicine*, 1996, Sept. 19, *335*(12), 966–969.

Cleveland, W. S. *The Elements of Graphing Data*. Monterey, Calif.: Wadsworth, 1985.

Demos, M. P., and Demos, N. P. "Statistical Quality Control's Role in Health Care Management." *Quality Progress*, 1989, *22*(8), 85–89.

Donabedian, A. *Explorations in Quality Assessment and Monitoring, Volume I: The Definition of Quality and Approaches to Its Assessment*. Ann Arbor, Mich.: Health Administration Press, 1980.

Donabedian, A. *Explorations in Quality Assessment and Monitoring, Volume II: The Criteria and Standards of Quality*. Ann Arbor, Mich.: Health Administration Press, 1982.

Donabedian, A. *Explorations in Quality Assessment and Monitoring, Volume III: The Methods and Findings of Quality Assessment: An Illustrated Analysis.* Ann Arbor, Mich.: Health Administration Press, 1985.

Epstein, A. M. "Definition, History, Scope and Characteristics of Physician Report Cards." In *Physician Assessment in the 21st Century: ABIM's Role.* Philadelphia: American Board of Internal Medicine, 1995.

Epstein, A. M. "Performance Reports on Quality: Prototypes, Problems and Prospects. *New England Journal of Medicine,* 1995, 333, 57–61.

Epstein, A. M. "The Role of Quality Measurement in a Competitive Marketplace." In S. Altman, U. Reinhardt (eds.), *Strategic Choices for a Changing Health Care System.* Chicago: Health Administration Press, 1996.

Green, J., and Wintfeld, N. "Report Cards on Cardiac Surgeons: Assessing New York State's Approach." *New England Journal of Medicine,* 1995, 332, 1229–1232.

Green, J., Wintfeld, N., Sharkey, P., and Passman, L. J. "The Importance of Severity of Illness in Assessing Hospital Mortality." *Journal of the American Medical Association,* 1990, 263, 241–246.

Hannan, E. L., Kilvurn, J. Jr., Bernard, H., O'Donnell, J. F. Lukacik, G., and Shields, E. P. "Coronary Artery Bypass Surgery: The Relationship Between In-Hospital Mortality Rate and Surgical Volume after Controlling for Clinical Risk Factors." *Medical Care,* 1991, 29, 1097–1107.

Hartert, T. V., Windom, H. H., Peebles, R. S., Freidhoff, L. R., and Togias, A. "Inadequate Outpatient Medical Yherapy for Patients with Asthma Admitted to Two Urban Hospitals." *American Journal of Medicine,* 1966, 100, 386–394.

Iezzoni, L. I. "Monitoring Quality of Care: What Do We Need to Know?" *Inquiry,* 1993, 30, 112–114.

Iezzoni, L. I., Ash, A. S., and Schwartz, M. "Judging Hospitals by Severity-Adjusted Mortality Rates: The Influence of the Severity-Adjusted Method." *American Journal of Public Health,* 1996, 86(10), 1379–1387.

Iezzoni, L. I., Restuccia, J. D., Shwartz, M., and others. "The Utility of Severity of Illness Information in Assessing the Quality of Hospital Care: The Role of the Clinical Trajectory." *Medical Care,* 1992, 30, 428–444.

Kassirer, J. P. "The Quality of Care and the Quality of Measuring it." *New England Journal of Medicine,* 1993, 329, 1263–1265.

Kazandjian, V. A., Thomson, R. G., Law, W. R. "Do Performance Indicators Make a Difference?" *The Joint Commission Journal on Quality Improvement,* 1997, 22(7), 482–483.

Leape, L. L., Park, R. E., Solomon, D. H., Chassin, M. R., Kisecoff, J., and
    Brook, R. H. "Does Inappropriate Use Explain Small Area Variations
    in the Use of Health Care Devices?" *Journal of the American Medical As-
    sociation*, 1994, *263*, 669–672.

Lesser, M. L., Robertson, S., and Kohn, N. "Statistical and Methodological
    Issues in the Evaluation of Care Management Studies." *Journal for Health-
    care Quality*, 1996, *18*(6): 25.

Murata, P. J., McGlynn, E. A., Siu, A. L., and others. "Quality Measures for Pre-
    natal Care: A Comparison of Care in Six Health Care Plans." *Archives of
    Family Medicine*, 1994, *3*, 41–49.

Nolan, T. W., and Provost, L. P. "Understanding Variation." *Quality Progress*,
    1990, May 1.

Report Card Pilot Project. *Key Findings and Lessons Learned: Twenty-One Plans'
    Performance Profiles*. Washington, D.C.: National Committee for Quality
    Assurance, 1995.

Rosen, L. S., Schroeder, K., and Hagan, M. "Adopting a Statewide Patient Data-
    base for Comparative Analysis and Quality Improvement." *Joint Commis-
    sion Journal on Quality Improvement*, 1996, *22*(7), 468–481.

Schneider, E. C., and Epstein, A. M. "Influence of Cardiac-Surgery Perfor-
    mance Reports on Referral Practices and Access to Care: A Survey of
    Cardiovascular Specialists." *New England Journal of Medicine*, 1996, *335*,
    251–256.

Sluyter, G. V., and Martin, M. A. "Measuring the Performance of Behavioral
    Health Care Organizations: A Proposed Model." *Best Practices and Bench-
    marking in Health Care*, 1996, *1*(6), 283.

Wakefield, D. S., Hendryx, M. S., and Uden-Holman, T. "Comparing Providers'
    Performance: Problems in Making the 'Report Card' Analogy Fit." *Journal
    for Healthcare Quality*, 1996, *18*.

Ware, J. E., Phillips, J., and Yody, B. B. "Assessment Tools: Functional Health
    Status and Patient Datisfaction." *American Journal of Medical Quality*,
    1996, *1*, S50–S53; *2*(1), S50–S53.

Wilson, A., and McDonald, P. "Comparison of Patient Questionnaire,
    Medical Record, and Audiotape in Assessment of Health Promotion
    in General Practice Consultations." *British Medical Journal*,1994, *309*,
    1483–1485.

Wilson, I. B., and Cleary, P. D. "Linking Clinical Variables with Health Related
    Quality of Life: A Conceptual Model of Patient Outcomes. *Journal of the
    American Medical Association*, 1995, *273*, 59–65.

## Guidelines, Protocols, Decision Support

Bassett, L. W., Hendrick, R. E., Bassford, T. L., and others. "Quality Determinants of Mammography." *Clinical Practice Guideline*, 13. Rockville, Md.: Department of Health and Human Services, 1994. (AHCPR publication no. 95–0632.)

Bergstrom, N., Allman, R. M., Alvarez, O. M., and others. "Treatment of Pressure Ulcers." *Clinical Practice Guideline*, 15. Rockville, Md.: Department of Health and Human Services, 1994. (AHCPR publication no. 95–0652.)

Bigos, S., Bowyer, O., Braen, G., and others. "Acute Low Back Problems in Adults." *Clinical Practice Guideline*, 14. Rockville, Md.: Department of Health and Human Services, 1994. (AHCPR publication no. 95–0642.)

Cataract Management Guideline Panel. "Cataract in Adults: Management of Functional Impairment." *Clinical Practice Guideline*, 4. Rockville, Md: Department of Health and Human Services, 1993. (AHCPR publication no. 93–0550.)

Depression Guideline Panel. *Depression in Primary Care. Vol. 1. Detection and Diagnosis. Clinical Practice Guideline*, 5. Rockville, Md.: Department of Health and Human Services, 1993. (AHCPR publication no. 93–0542.)

Eccles, M., Clapp, Z., Grimshaw, J., and others. "North of England Evidence Based Guidelines Development Project: Methods of Guideline Development." *British Medical Journal*, 1996, *312*, 760–762.

El-Sadr, W., Oleske, J. M., Agins, B. D., and others. "Evaluation and Management of Early HIV Infection." *Clinical Practice Guideline*, 7. Rockville, Md.: Department of Health and Human Services, 1994. (AHCPR publication no. 94–0572.)

Fink, A., Kosecoff, J., Chassin, M., and Brook, R. H. "Consensus Methods: Characteristics and Guidelines for Use." *American Journal of Public Health*, 1984, *74*, 979–983.

Greireder, D. K. "The Adoption of Asthma Practice Guidelines into Clinical Care: The Harvard Pilgrim Health Care Experience." *The Journal of Outcomes Management*, 1996, *3*(3): 9.

Grimshaw, J. M., and Russell, I. T. "Effect of Clinical Guidelines on Medical Practice: A Systematic Review of Rigorous Evaluations." *Lancet* 1993, *342*, 1317–1322.

Hickey, M. L., Kleefield, S. F., and Pearson, S. D. "Payor-Hospital Collaboration to Improve Patient Satisfaction with Hospital Discharge." *The Joint Commission Journal on Quality Improvement*, 1996, *22*(5), 336–344.

James, B. C. "Implementing Practice Guidelines Through Clinical Quality Improvement." *Frontiers in Health Service Management*, 1993, *10*(1), 3–37.

"Key Findings and Lessons Learned: Twenty-One Plans' Performance Profiles." *NCQA Technical Report*. Washington D.C.: Report Card Pilot Project, 1993.

Konstam, M. A., Dracup, K., Baker, D. W., and others. "Heart Failure: Evaluation and Care of Patients with Left-Ventricular Systolic Dysfunction." *Clinical Practice Guideline*, 11. Rockville, Md.: Department of Health and Human Services, 1994. (AHCPR publication no. 94–0612.)

McConnell, J. D., Barry, M. J., Bruskewitz, R. C., and others. "Benign Prostatic Hyperplasia: Diagnosis and Treatment." *Clinical Practice Guideline*, 8. Rockville, Md.: Department of Health and Human Services, 1994. (AHCPR publication no. 94–0582.)

Moore, M. "A New Approach to Clinical Decision Support." *Medical Practice Management*, 1997, March/April, 249–253.

Morrell, C., Harvey, G., and Kitson, A. "Practitioner-Based Quality Improvement: A Review of the Royal College of Nursing's Dynamic Standard Setting System. *Quality in Health Care*, 1997, 6(1), 29–34.

North of England Asthma Guideline Development Group. "North of England Evidence Based Guidelines Development Project: Summary Version of Evidence Based Guideline for the Primary Care Management of Asthma in Adults." *British Medical Journal*, 1996, *312*, 762–766.

North of England Stable Angina Guideline Development Group. "North of England Evidence Based Guidelines Development Project: Summary Version of Evidence Based Guideline for the Primary Care Management of Stable Angina." *British Medical Journal*, 1996, *312*, 827–832.

Pestonik, S. L., Classen, D. C., Evans, R. S., and Burke, J. P. "Implementing Antibiotic Practice Guidelines Through Computer-Assisted Decision Support: Clinical Outcomes and Financial Outcomes. *Annals of Internal Medicine*, 1996, *124*, 884–890.

"Phone Treatment Protocols for Common Minor Medical Complaints." *Eye on Improvement*, June 1, 1997.

Sickle Cell Disease Guideline Panel. "Sickle Cell Disease: Screening, Diagnosis, Management, and Counseling in Newborns and Infants." *Clinical Practice Guideline*, 6. Rockville, Md.: Department of Health and Human Services, 1993. (AHCPR publication no. 93–0562.)

Stool, S. E., Berg, A. O., Berman, S., and others. "Otitis Media with Effusion in Young Children." *Clinical Practice Guideline*, 12. Rockville, Md.: Department of Health and Human Services, 1993. (AHCPR publication no. 94–0622.)

Studnicki, J., Remmell, R., and Campbell, R. "The Impact of Legislatively Imposed Practice Guidelines on Cesarean Section Rates: The Florida Experience." *American Journal of Medical Quality*, 1997, *12*(1), 62.

Wenger, N. K., Froelicher, E. S., Smith, L. K., and others. "Cardiac Rehabilitation." *Clinical Practice Guideline*, 17. Rockville, Md.: Department
of Health and Human Services, 1994. (AHCPR publication no.
96–0672.)

# Managed Care Issues

Berwick, D. M. "Payment by Capitation and the Quality of Care." *New England
Journal of Medicine*, 1996, *335*(16), 1227–1230.

Carey, T. S., and Weis, K. "Diagnostic Testing and Return Visits for Acute Problems in Prepaid, Case-Managed Medicaid Plans Compared with Fee-for-
Service." *Archives in Internal Medicine*, 1990, *150*, 2369–2372.

Carey, T. S., Weis, K., and Homer, C. "Prepaid versus Traditional Medicaid
Plans: Effects on Preventive Health Care." *Journal of Clinical Epidemiology*,
1990, *43*, 1213–1220.

Carey, T. S., Weis, K, and Homer, C. "Prepaid versus Traditional Medicaid
Plans: Lack of Effect on Pregnancy Outcomes and Prenatal Care." *Health
Services Research*, 1991, 26:165–181.

Carlisle, D. M., Siu, A. L., Keeler, E. B., and others. "HMO vs. Fee-for-Service
Care of Older Persons with Acute Myocardial Infarction." *American Journal of Public Health*, 1992, *82*, 1626–1630.

Cigich, S. M., and Mischler, N. E. "Success in Managed Care: Improving Clinical Quality." *The Physician Executive*, 1997, April, 24–31.

Clement, D. G., Tetchin, S. M., Brown, R. S., and Stegall, M. H. "Access and
Outcomes of Elderly Patients Enrolled in Managed Care." *Journal of the
American Medical Association*, 1994, *271*, 1487–1492. [Erratum, 1994,
*272*, 276.]

Gold, M. R., Hurley, R., Lake, T., Ensor, T., and Berenson, R. "A National Survey of the Arrangements Managed Care Plans Make with Physicians."
*New England Journal of Medicine*, 1995, *333*, 1678–1683.

Goldfarb, S. "Physicians in Control of the Capitated Dollar: Do unto Others. . . ."
*Annals of Internal Medicine*, 1995, *123*, 546–547.

"HCFA Weights Shift to Patient Outcomes as Key to Hospital Medicare Eligi-
bility." *Physician Manager*, 1997, 8(5), 1.

HEDIS 3.0 Draft for Public Comment. Health Plan Employer Data and Information Set. Washington, D.C.: National Committee for Quality Assurance,
July 1996.

Hillman, A. L. "Financial Incentives for Physicians in HMOs: Is There a
Conflict of Interest?" New England Journal of Medicine, 1987, *317*,
1743–1748.

Hillman, A. L. "Managing the Physician: Rules Versus Incentives." *Health Affairs* (Millwood) 1991, *10*(4), 138–146.

Hillman, A. L., Pauly, M. V., Kerman, K., and Martinck, C. R. "HMO Managers' Views on Financial Incentives and Quality." *Health Affairs* (Millwood) 1991, *10*(4), 207–219.

Hillman, A. L., Pauly, M. V., Kerstein, J. J. "How Do Financial Incentives Affect Physicians' Clinical Decisions and the Financial Performance of Health Maintenance Organization?" *New England Journal of Medicine*, 1989, *321*, 86–92.

Lurie, N., Christianson, J. B., Finch, M., and Moscovice, I. "The Effects of Capitation on Health and Functional Status of the Medicaid Elderly: A Randomized Trial." *Annals of Internal Medicine*, 1994, *120*, 506–511.

Lurie, N., Moscovice, I. S., Finch, M., Christianson, J. B., and Popkin, M. K. "Does Capitation Affect the Health of the Chronically Mentally Ill? Results from a Randomized Trial." *Journal of the American Medical Association*, 1992, *267*, 3300–3304.

"Managing Congestive Heart Failure Care Critical for Medicare Risk Contracting." *Physician Manager*, 1997, 8(4), 1, 8.

Murray, J. P., Greenfield, S., Kaplan, S. H., and Yano, E. M. "Ambulatory Testing for Capitation and Fee-for-Service Patients in the Same Practice Setting: Relationship to Outcomes." *Medical Care*, 1992, *30*, 252–261.

Retchin, S. M., and Brown, B. "Management of Colorectal Cancer in Medicare Health Maintenance Organizations." *Journal of General Internal Medicine*, 1990, *5*, 110–114.

Retchin, S. M., and Brown, B. "The Quality of Ambulatory Care in Medicare Health Maintenance Organizations." *American Journal of Public Health*, 1990, *80*, 411–415.

Retchin, S. M., and Brown, B. "Elderly Patients with Congestive Heart Failure under Prepaid Care." *American Journal of Medicine*, 1991, *90*, 236–242.

Ware, J. E. Jr., Brook, R. H., Rogers, W. H., and others. "Comparison of Health Outcomes at a Health Maintenance Organization with Those of Fee-for-Service Care." *Lancet* 1986, *1*, 1017–1022.

# Redesigning the Delivery of Care

Barbret, L. C., Wesphal, C. G., and Daly, G. A. "Meeting Information Needs of Families of Critical Care Patients." *Journal for Healthcare Quality*, 1997, *19*(2), 5–10.

Cohen, B. A., Grigonis, A. M., and Topper, M. E. "The Development of an Out-comes Management System for Acute Medical Rehabilitation." *American Journal of Medical Quality*, 1997, *12*(1), 28–32.

Gerteis, M., Edgman-Levitan, S., Daley, J., and Delbanco, T. L. (eds.). *Through the Patient's Eyes: Understanding and Promoting Patient Centered Care*. San Francisco: Jossey-Bass, 1993.

Hacquebord H. "Health Care from the Perspective of the Patient: Theories for Improvement." *Quality Management in Health Care* 1994, *2*(2), 68–75.

Kazandjian, V. A., Thomson, R. G., and Law, W. R. "Do Performance Indicators Make a Difference?" *The Joint Commission Journal on Quality Improvement*, 1997, *22*(7), 482–483.

Kelly, D. L., Pestorik, S. L., and Coons, M. C. "Reengineering a Surgical Service Line: Focusing on Core Process Improvement." *American Journal of Medical Quality*, 1997, *12*(2), 120–129.

Lahdensuo, A., Haahtela, T., Herrala, J., and others. "Randomized Comparison of Guided Self-Management and Traditional Treatment of Asthma over One Year." *British Medical Journal*, 1996, *312*, 748–752.

Maurana, C. A., Langley, A. E., and Goldberg, K. "Applying TQM to an Academic Partnership." *Quality Digest*, 1997, September, 50–54.

"Mayo Medical Center Improves Telephone Access in Referring Physician Service." *Eye on Improvement*, July 1, 1997.

"Medical Associates Improves Specialty Referral Process." *Eye on Improvement*, March 15, 1997.

"Re-engineering Support Services." *Eye on Improvement*, February 15, 1997.

"Re-engineering the ICU Utilizing TQM Principles." *Eye on Improvement*, January 15, 1997.

Welch, H. G., Wennberg, D. E., and Welch, W. P. "The Use of Medicare Home Health Care Services." *New England Journal of Medicine*, 1996, *335*(5), 324–329.

Ziegler, J. "The Mind, the Body, and the Benefits Budget." *Business and Health*, 1997, *15*(2), 22–28.

## Building Teams and Leadership in the Organization

Antai-Ontong, D. "Team Building in a Health Care Setting: What It Means to be a Good Team Player—and How You Can be Most Effective on Your Health Care Team." *American Journal of Nursing* 1997, *97*(7), 48–51.

Davis, D. A., Thomson, M. A., Oxman, A. D., and Haynes, R. B. "Changing Physician Performance: A Systematic Review of the Effect of Continuing

Medical Education Strategies." *Journal of the American Medical Association*, 1995, *274*, 700–705.

Harper, A., and Harper, B. *Team Barriers: Actions for Overcoming the Blocks to Empowerment, Involvement, and High Performance*. New York: MW Corporation, 1994.

Kleeb, T. E. "Collaboration: A Framework for Clinical Quality Improvement." *Journal for Healthcare Quality*, 1997, *19*(4), 10–17.

Marszalek-Gaucher, E., and Coffey, R. J. *Transforming Healthcare Organizations: How to Achieve and Sustain Organizational Excellence*. San Francisco: Jossey-Bass, 1990.

McCorcle M. D., and Heet, N. S. "The 'Success Test': Validating the Competencies Required for Healthcare Leadership." *Best Practices and Benchmarking in Healthcare*, 1997, *2*(2), 63–70.

Prather, S. E., Blake, R. R., and Mouton, J. S. *Behavioral Types and the Art of Patient Management*. Los Angeles: Practice Management Information Corp., 1995.

Scholtes, P. R. *The Team Handbook: How to Use Teams to Improve Quality*. Madison, Wis.: Joiner Associates, 1988.

# Index

Printed and bound by CPI Group (UK) Ltd, Croydon, CR0 4YY

16/04/2025

14658442-0006